An Ounce of Prevention

"The first wealth is health"

– Ralph Waldo Emerson

PLEASE READ THE DISCLAIMER CAREFULLY BEFORE USING THIS BOOK

This book is for educational purposes only. It is not intended to diagnose, treat, or cure any disease. Remember each person's body is different and may react differently to various supplements and therapies. Use the information found in this book as precisely that: Information. This information is not meant to replace a medical consultation and is not a substitute for your personal physician's advice. You and your doctor must make any final decisions.

An Ounce *of* Prevention

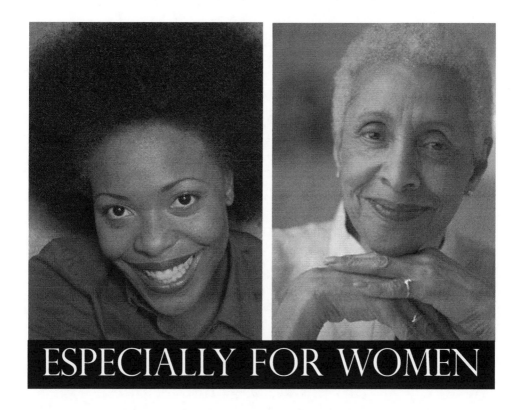

ESPECIALLY FOR WOMEN

Dr Anthony Vendryes

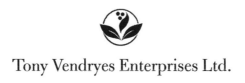

Tony Vendryes Enterprises Ltd.

First published in Jamaica 2010 by
Tony Vendryes Enterprises Ltd.
P. O. Box 195
Montego Bay, St James
Jamaica W.I.

E-mail: drvendryes@gmail.com

www.anounceofprevention.org

© 2010 by Dr Anthony Vendryes.

All rights reserved. No part of this publication may be reproduced or
transmitted in any form or by any means, electronic or mechanical,
including photocopying, recording or any information storage and
retrieval system without the written permission of the author.

ISBN: 978-976-610-811-3

A catalogue record of this book is available
from the National Library of Jamaica.

Cover and book design by Robert Harris
(email: roberth@cwjamaica.com)

Cover photograph of Dr Anthony Vendryes by Michael Chen.

Set in Bulmer Mt Regular 12.5/16 x 30

Printed in the United States of America.

This book is dedicated to
all the women of the world especially those who
have personally enriched my life: my mother Maria, my wife Dorothy,
my sisters, aunts, nieces and other female family members,
friends, staff, business associates and patients.

Thank you for your feminine energy, your love, your wisdom and
your inspiration. May the information I share in this book, in some
small way express my gratitude to you.

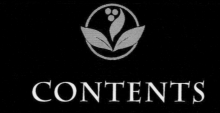

CONTENTS

SECTION 1:   WELLNESS CONCEPTS / 1

SECTION 2:   HEALTHY AGENTS & PRACTICES / 21

SECTION 4:   FEMALE ISSUES / 159

SECTION 5:   DANGER AREAS / 205

SECTION 6:   WEIGHT MANAGEMENT / 251

APPENDICES / 277

D r Vendryes' first book *An Ounce of Prevention: New and Natural Ways to Prevent Common Health Problems* has been at my desk for the last six years. It has served as a reference to counsel and guide my patients as they use herbs, nutrition and botanicals for their health. I felt it was almost like having a full time consultant in the office.

When I first heard of a second book, I actually was not sure I needed it. I therefore waited in anticipation for a draft to review before I passed judgment as to a need for another book.

I was taken aback by the incredible addition that this new book brings to me personally and to my thousands of patients. If it was possible to improve on the first book, this book exceeded all my expectations!

Dr Vendryes has an uncanny ability to communicate in clear, precise, uncomplicated terms as he guides the reader through a topic. This clarity sets this book apart from others, which address similar topics.

Through radio, private consultations, public lectures and the written word, Dr Vendryes has profoundly affected thousands of lives. This new book adds one more chapter in his life of dedication to serving mankind and making the world a place where self-care and personal acceptance of health decisions draws together the wisdom of the past and the future course of health and wellness.

It is with no hesitation that I recommend this new book to all who care about quality of life, natural physiology, and the innate ability for our bodies to be healthy and well if given the proper nutrition and balanced with the gifts of botanicals.

Thank you Dr Vendryes for once again filling a need for more light and knowledge regarding these complex bodies we live in!

Steven A. Komadina, MD, FACOG, Director Health Horizons Lifestyle Medicine,
Past President New Mexico Medical Society,
New Mexico State Senator 2001–2009

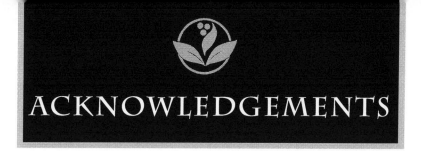

ACKNOWLEDGEMENTS

The overwhelmingly positive response to my first book, *An Ounce of Prevention: New and Natural Ways to Prevent Common Health Problems,* along with the ever-expanding body of new and useful information on human health have been major catalysts for the writing of this book.

To the many individuals who contributed to its creation, I say thank you. To my wise and ever supportive project manager and publisher Robert Harris, and Lisa Morgan my efficient editor, thanks for enduring all my changes and delays. It has been a pleasure and a privilege working with you all.

To the editor and staff of the Gleaner Company and the Management and staff of POWER106FM, I thank you for allowing the message of this book to be already read and heard all over the world in print and on air.

My thanks to that vast number of medical researchers worldwide, who continue to document and report on the amazing ability of the human body, mind and spirit to heal itself.

To my wife Dorothy, other family members, staff, inner circle of friends, my mentors and coaches, thank you for believing in me and my message. With very special gratitude and joy, I thank my spiritual Guru, Yogi Amrit Desai, for his love, his guidance and his grace.

Finally, to the Divine, from whom all blessings flow, I thank you my God!

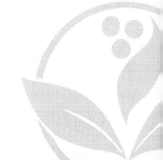

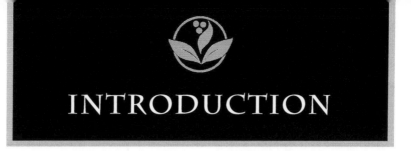

INTRODUCTION

'Maintaining order rather than correcting disorder is the
ultimate principle of wisdom. To cure disease after it has appeared
is like digging a well when one is already thirsty, or forging
weapons after the war has already begun.'

– Chinese Emperor Huang Ti (Second century BC)

An Ounce of Prevention, is subtitled 'Especially for Women' for several reasons. Over two thirds of the people who seek my advice are women: they are the majority of my patients. Also, the woman in a household has a potentially very powerful influence on the lifestyle of all who live there. She is usually the one who controls the kitchen and the food, who does the grocery shopping and sets the tone for the lifestyle habits of the entire family. So, in focusing on women, I seek to speak to the entire family, community and nation.

In addition, women have a number of unique health problems. It is not without significance that an entire specialty in medicine – Gynaecology – is devoted to the treatment of female disorders. But, our women are suffering unnecessarily and dying prematurely from conditions that are eminently preventable and often correctable with relatively simple approaches. This message needs to be heard.

This book, like its predecessor, is a compilation of articles published each week in the *Daily Gleaner*, Jamaica's oldest and largest newspaper. Each chapter is an article covering a specific issue in a short easy to read format. My intention is that, in a few minutes, the reader will understand the approach I have to a specific condition or problem and the simple action plan of how to deal with it.

Some of the chapters from the previous book have been revised while others have been omitted to make room for new material. An entire section has been devoted to specific female issues while the other sections cover topics of relevance to man, woman and child.

I consider myself a 'Medical Maverick' and have often been asked by my patients 'What do your medical colleagues think of your different methods?' I can answer in the words of a 17th century English physician, himself a medical maverick:

> It is my nature to think where others read, to ask less whether the world agrees with me, than whether I agree with the truth, and to hold cheap the rumour and applause of the multitude. (Thomas Sydenham, 1624–1689)

I hope that in reading this book many will be empowered to take action to prevent and reverse these common disorders, and so live healthier and happier lives. Notwithstanding the book disclaimer the approaches described here represents the actual recommendations that I make to my own patients. Remember, 'Your health is in your hands. Treat it with care and handle it with love.'

TONY VENDRYES, MB, BS, DA, FRCA

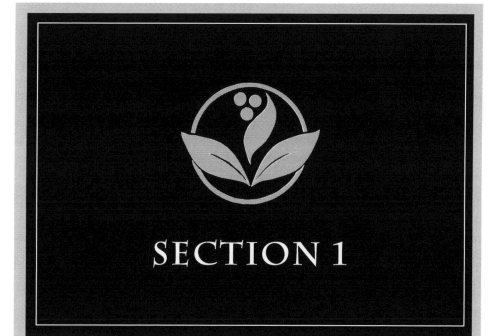

SECTION 1

WELLNESS
CONCEPTS

*'Everyone has a doctor in him or her; we just
have to help it in its work. The natural healing force
within each one of us is the greatest force in getting well.'*

– Hippocrates, Greek physician (460 BC–377 BC)

www.anounceofprevention.org

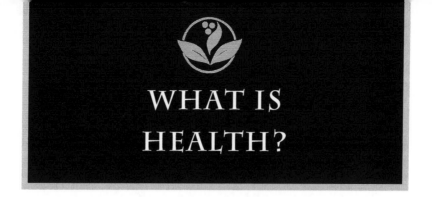

WHAT IS HEALTH?

'Health is a state of complete physical, mental and social wellbeing, and not merely the absence of disease or infirmity.'
– World Health Organization, 1948

My own belief is that the human body was designed to be healthy. When the good book says that we are fearfully and wonderfully made, it is not just a nice sounding phrase; it is really true. The human body has an incredible capacity to heal and repair itself. Illness and disease are a reflection of our failure to take proper care of our bodies and minds.

As a doctor, I have come to understand that I cannot really heal anyone. Healing is something that happens from within. Your body is the healer and the doctor's role is to provide the support and assistance to facilitate the healing process. Until we, as a society, fully accept this concept, we will continue to face the dilemma of 'more medicines, less health'.

FOUR PILLARS OF WELLNESS

From my experience, there are four basic concepts that underpin and support real health. I call them the Four Pillars of Wellness. These are:

- Nutrition
- Exercise
- Detoxification
- Stress management

These four simple but powerful processes form the basis of my approach to virtually all the common lifestyle related disorders that comprise health.

Nutrition

This is the first and probably the most critical pillar, because you literally are what you eat. Your body is composed of trillions of cells – the building blocks of the body. Your body is constantly repairing and renewing itself, as each day millions of old damaged cells die and new ones are created to replace them. Your body is a work in progress.

But the quality and vitality of the new cells being created in your body right now, as you read this chapter, depends on the quality of the food you have been eating. Garbage in will produce garbage out. Medical experts believe that as much as two thirds of today's health problems are related to our unhealthy diet.

For almost 15 years, I have used and recommended a concept and program called Cellular Nutrition for my patients and myself to enjoy the best nutrition. The idea is simple: give the cells of the body the nutrients that they need and they will know how to heal, mend and repair. It works!

Exercise

As the old saying goes: use it or lose it. The human body can be compared to a high performance car. It needs high quality fuel in the gas tank. That's the nutritional part. But the body is designed to be active. If you never drove your car and left it parked all the time, the engine would eventually seize up and the body begin to rust away.

Similarly, many people are in fact suffering from 'seize up' and 'rust down' because of inactivity. Muscles get weak, joints get stiff, heart and lungs lose their efficiency, and tension and stress overwhelm your mind. The research shows that as little as 20 to 30 minutes of exercise, three to four times per week can result in amazing benefits to your physical and mental health.

Detoxification

Not only do we live in a polluted world with chemicals and impurities in the food we eat, the water we drink and bathe in and the air we breathe, but just as a car engine produces toxic exhaust fumes, so the body's metabolism produces toxic wastes. Sadly, the body's natural pathways for elimination of these poisons are often blocked and function poorly. We all carry a toxic burden.

The body normally detoxifies itself via the bowels, the liver, the kidneys, the skin and breath. Several simple natural techniques are available to assist the body to get rid of accumulated impurities. These are referred to as cleansing or detoxification programs.

Stress management

Stress is a poorly understood concept. It is not a thing or person or circumstance. Those 'things' are called stressors. Stress is a reaction – your internal reaction – to the stressor. Understanding this is critical because, often, we cannot change or stressors, for example, our spouse or boss, but we can always learn to change the way we reduce them. In essence, stress management is self-management.

Sadly, many so-called stress management programs really focus on stressor management. Real stress management is a skill that can be taught and learnt, just like how we can learn to swim or ride a bicycle. Stress is indeed the enemy within!

So, make your Four Pillars of Wellness strong and solid and you will enjoy true health and wellness.

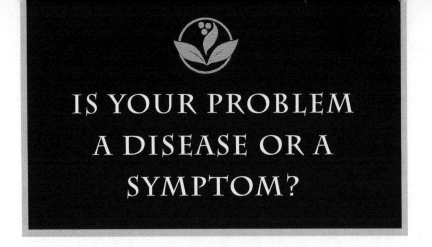

IS YOUR PROBLEM A DISEASE OR A SYMPTOM?

'Symptoms, then, are in reality nothing but the cry from suffering organs.'
– Jean Martin Charcot

Ask yourself this question: Is an elevation of your blood cholesterol level or your blood sugar level or your blood pressure level or your body temperature a disease or really a symptom or sign of some underlying problem? I believe that the answer is that these are symptoms. They are like signposts warning us that there is some deeper disorder to be addressed.

If this is in fact true, then much of conventional medical efforts to treat these common issues are about symptom management, usually with a pill, with little attention to the root problem. If there were a flood in your house, would you first reach for the mop before turning off the tap? No, that would seem insane. So, is our so-called 'Health Care System' also insane?

BIGPHARM

No, our Sickness Care System is not insane. It is simply being manipulated by one of the greatest economic forces in the world – the Pharmaceutical Industry aka 'BIGPHARM'. This is the power that controls, manipulates and directs the way medical care is delivered. To give some indication of their power, in 1995 it was reported that on the Fortune 500 (the 500 most profitable companies on Wall Street), the total profits of the top eight drug companies was more than the combined profits of the other 492 companies. That is **POWER**. That is **INFLUENCE**. That is **CONTROL**.

This industry determines how medical research is carried out, what drugs are developed, how doctors are trained and how patients are treated. Is there a legal drug cartel? There is nothing wrong with these companies making a profit, but what if the price we pay is too high?

A HIGH PRICE TO PAY

The current drug based health care system is too expensive. The economies of affluent countries like the US and Britain are burdened by the cost of their health care models. A prominent economist recently suggested that the thing most likely to cripple the US economy is the cost of its health care system. The US government will not be able to afford the spiralling cost of Medicare and Medicaid. Too much of its budget is being spent on health care. This is apart from what people themselves pay for health insurance and doctors' fees. What about a country like Jamaica? Can we afford to be using such a system?

A DANGEROUS WAY TO GO

The well-researched documentary, *Prescription for Disaster*, reveals that the number one cause of death in the United States today is doctoring! Doctor-prescribed medication and medical treatments now kill more Americans than any other single agent. Is this the model that Jamaica should be imitating?

The number of drugs that have to be withdrawn from the market because of adverse side effects is most alarming. Even more distressing is the evidence that, in many instances, the drug companies knew about these side effects and manipulated the research results so that the drug would still be sold to the gullible public by misinformed or indifferent doctors.

Only after the death, suffering and distress of the patients became too great to ignore, would the authorities apologetically withdraw the drug and the drug companies be allowed to make off with their huge bloodstained profits. In the language of warfare, they write the suffering off as 'colateral damage'. The arthritis drug VIOXX® is only one example of this phenomenon. On September 30, 2004, Merck voluntarily withdrew VIOXX® from the market because of concerns about increased risk of heart attack and stroke associated with long-term, high-dosage use.

Yes, modern medicine has developed wonderful technologies for treating many acute problems. I recognise and applaud these. If I am injured in an accident, I will be heading for the hospital. But the fact is that most of today's major health problems are chronic, lifestyle-related disorders. These require the coaching, training and motivation of our people in lifestyle and behaviour modification, not drugs and surgery. The answers to these health issues are often found in simple things like nutrition, exercise and stress management.

Obesity, high blood pressure, blood sugar imbalance, high cholesterol levels, and so on, are mostly indicators that we need to change our lifestyle. Drugs to lower cholesterol, control blood sugar, reduce blood pressure or gastric bypass surgery to treat obesity should be reserved for rare, exceptional circumstances. Instead these drugs and procedures are being promoted more and more as a first line response. Madness!

So why are we doing this madness? This madness makes some people rich. You find the answer by following the money trail. That is the problem.

THE ANSWER

The present situation will not change by itself. BIGPHARM will not surrender its profits and I fear that, sadly, the medical profession has surrendered its moral authority and power to create change. The change will have to come from the patient, the public, the consumer – you and mavericks like me.

We are actually the ones with the power. We are the ones who decide how we spend our money, what kind of doctor we consult and what we choose to take or not take. We can demand a different approach, but we must inform ourselves about our choices. Sometimes the conventional approach may be appropriate and at other times it may not. We must make informed decisions.

The change is in fact happening. Back in 1991, the *New England Journal of Medicine* reported that more Americans chose alternative health care than conventional medicine, even though they had to pay out of pocket as their insurance companies did not cover those therapies.

On a daily basis I am approached by people who refuse to accept the advice that their only option is to take this or that drug for the rest of their lives. Something deep inside resists the idea that their problem is incurable and that they can only control their symptoms with drugs. They are tired of just using the mop. They want to try to turn off the tap. They want to get to the root of their problem. They want to take more responsibility for their health.

I champion and promote that thinking. Whatever empowers the individual, I support. Whatever is disempowering and makes a person feel like a helpless victim, I strongly question. Let us all make a commitment to be a part of the solution and not just 'hug up' the problem. Let us reduce the attention on sickness management and let's really emphasise prevention, healthy lifestyles and wellness.

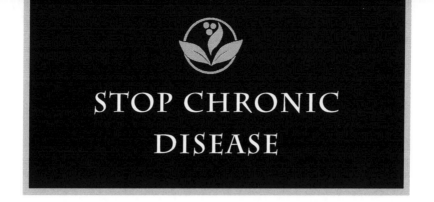

STOP CHRONIC DISEASE

*"If I knew that I would live this long, I would
have taken better care of myself"*
– Woody Allen

Many of our commonest illnesses are called chronic degenerative diseases. Why? Because they develop slowly, over many years, from abuse and poor care but end up causing severe pain, suffering and even death. In effect, our bodies degenerate because of the way we treat them.

The undeniable medical evidence is that poor nutrition and bad lifestyle choices during childhood predispose us to these debilitating degenerative diseases later in life. Examples of these diseases include heart disease, cancer, osteoporosis, diabetes and hypertension.

FOCUS ON WHAT YOU EAT

Medical research has established an indisputable link between nutrition and health. Literally hundreds of scientific studies have indicated a strong association between diet and the incidence of chronic degenerative disease. We know, for example, that by eating a varied and balanced diet that is low in saturated fat and rich in fruits, vegetables, and complex carbohydrates (particularly fibre), we can reduce the risk of heart disease, cancer, and Type II diabetes. Diets rich in tomato products containing lycopene are known to reduce the incidence of prostate cancer in men. And diets rich in green leafy vegetables, particularly those containing lutein, are associated with reducing the risk of macular degeneration, a common cause of blindness.

TAKE VITAMINS AND MINERALS

Further research has linked the intake of certain vitamins and minerals to long-term health. Vitamin E supplements (400–800 IU per day) are linked to a reduction of heart disease. Calcium and vitamin D are known to reduce bone loss and the risk of osteoporosis in post-menopausal women. Folic acid, vitamin B_{12} and vitamin B_6 can lower blood homocysteine, a risk factor for heart disease.

In short, good nutrition – achieved through a balanced diet and supplementing with optimal levels of appropriate vitamins and minerals – is critical for preventing these chronic illnesses.

START EARLY

Medical evidence shows that chronic degenerative diseases are not necessarily diseases of old age. Their beginnings are often evident in children, adolescents, and young adults. Here are some examples:

Heart disease

We know that heart disease starts in childhood. A recent article published in the *New England Journal of Medicine* shows the beginnings of heart disease in children 2–15 years old. The study further reported that the prevalence of heart disease increases with age, affecting about 30 percent of adolescents 16–20 years old, 50 per cent of young adults 21–25 years old, and 70 per cent of adults 26–39 years old.

Other research shows that:

- 30–40 percent of heart disease deaths directly result from obesity.
- Childhood obesity doubles the risk of adult obesity.
- The most effective strategy for preventing heart disease in adulthood is to prevent obesity in childhood. Unfortunately, more Jamaican children are overweight today than ever before.

Cancer

Most cancers take decades to develop before they are diagnosed. Our cells have many safeguards against cancerous proliferation, and it generally takes tens of years for enough genetic damage to accumulate to override all the safe-guards. Once a cell becomes cancerous, it can take decades more before a tumour is detected. Because we estimate that 30–35 per cent of all cancers are related to diet, we can logically assume that childhood diet plays a significant role in defining adult cancer risk, and growing medical evidence supports this assumption.

Osteoporosis

Osteoporosis is a degenerative disease tied to poor nutrition during early years. Epidemiological studies show that maintaining good calcium nutrition and attaining high bone mineral density during adolescence lead both to improved bone mineral density and to reduced risk of osteoporosis later in life. In fact, it is estimated that adolescent girls who increase bone mass by as little as 5 percent during their teen years can reduce the risk of osteoporosis after menopause by 40 per cent.

THE BOTTOM LINE

The essential point is that good nutrition is a lifelong imperative. To optimize our health over a lifetime, we must optimize nutrition during all stages of life. The time to eat well and practise good nutritional habits is now, whether we are 4, 14, 34, or 64 years old. It is essential that we teach our children how to eat today to prevent the chronic degenerative diseases of tomorrow.

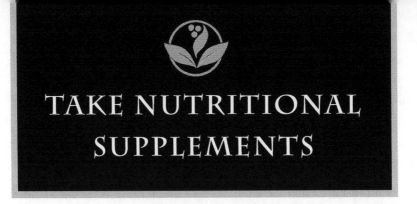

TAKE NUTRITIONAL SUPPLEMENTS

'Of several remedies, the physician should choose the least sensational.'
– Hippocrates

Up until the end of the last century, mainstream medicine was openly hostile to the idea of healthy people taking vitamin supplements. Only recently has this anti-vitamin position begun to change, as irrefutable evidence emerged showing that vitamin supplements could reduce the risk of many common diseases. Sadly, it is still common practice for doctors to tell their patients that they do not need vitamin supplements if they are eating a 'balanced' diet.

In April 1998, the editorial in the *New England Journal of Medicine* was entitled 'Eat Right and Take a Multi-Vitamin'. This article indicated that certain vitamin supplements could reduce the risk of heart attacks and strokes. This was the first time that a prestigious medical journal was recommending vitamin supplements.

An even stronger endorsement for the use of vitamin supplements came in the June 19, 2002 issue of the *Journal of the American Medical Association*. Harvard University doctors reported that people who got enough vitamins might be able to prevent such common illnesses as cancer, heart disease and osteoporosis.

Today nearly 35 per cent of North Americans take multivitamins but many are reluctant to tell their doctors for fear that they may disapprove. I suspect that the same situation exists right here in Jamaica, although I have observed that a number of my Jamaican medical colleagues are now recommending vitamin and herbal supplements to their patients. I applaud them.

However, to confuse the issue, research suggests that as much as one third of dietary supplements (vitamins, minerals and herbals), mostly imported from the United States have one or all of the following problems:

- The products do not contain what the label says it should.

- The products contain other undisclosed substances in addition to what is on the label, which may create a health hazard.

- The active ingredients in a supplement may not be readily absorbed by the system, and may thus be ineffective.

Fortunately, the Jamaican Ministry of Health is currently seeking to find ways to protect the interests of the public in this matter. I hope, however, that in doing so the right of the individual to choose supplements for himself or herself will not be infringed upon. After all, the possible problems that may arise from taking supplements are minute when compared with the side effects of prescription medication. Just imagine, over 150,000 Americans die each year from the side effects of drugs prescribed by their doctors!

HOW TO CHOOSE AND USE NUTRITIONAL SUPPLEMENTS

The following guidelines will help you in your choice and use of nutritional supplements.

Choose a reputable brand

The cheapest brand is not necessarily the best. Choose products from a company that has an established reputation for high quality and effective products. Speak with individuals who have used that brand and have them share their experience with you. Well-trained network marketers of nutritional supplements are particularly helpful in this regard, as they are usually heavy consumers of the products they sell. Some, but not all, health food store personnel may also be helpful. I myself very carefully select the brand of supplements I recommend to my clients.

Read the labels

The US Food and Drug Administration monitors and regulates dietary supplements using two main laws:

1. The Megadosage Law, which says that no food supplement should have an amount of any one ingredient that could create harm when taken at the recommended dosage.

2. The Labeling Law, which says that any potential side effect that a dietary supplement may have and any necessary warnings about the use of such a product should appear on the product's label.

Unfortunately, unscrupulous manufacturers often get away with outright fraud and that is why my first recommendation is so important.

Pay little attention to RDA (Recommended Daily Allowance) values on the labels. The RDA is the minimum amount of a vitamin necessary to prevent you from being seriously deficient. I believe that those levels are far too low for optimal health benefits. In fact, many experts believe that the RDA is obsolete and irrelevant to modern nutritional practice.

Educate yourself

The more informed you become about nutrition, the more responsibility you can take for maintaining excellent health. There are many books, tapes, seminars and Internet sites that provide good information. I recommend my own book, *An Ounce of Prevention*, as a good information source. Remember, 'Your Health is in your Hands'.

Talk with your doctor

It is important that your doctor knows that you are taking supplements. If your doctor is unwilling to discuss the matter with you, then I would suggest that you seek a second opinion or even change your health care provider. Remember, doctors are often not well educated about nutrition and nutritional supplementation.

Balance your nutrition

Despite their importance, multivitamin tablets alone are not a replacement for a balanced, healthy diet. They should complement your diet. Particularly try to have at least seven servings of fresh fruits and vegetables daily. These contain a variety of beneficial substances, known and unknown. Try to include a high quality nutritional protein shake drink in your daily diet. Remember, good Cellular Nutrition is basic to good health.

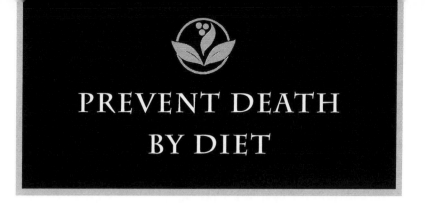

PREVENT DEATH BY DIET

'If in doubt, try nutrition first.'
– Roger J. Williams

The news is full of reports these days on the relationship between health and diet, between illness and food. Finally the message seems to be getting through – we are digging our graves with our teeth. Over 70 per cent of all deaths this year will be due to only three conditions:

- Heart disease
- Cancer
- Stroke (caused by diabetes and high blood pressure)

All these diseases have one thing in common – they are nutritionally-related disorders. The most important risk factor for these diseases is not your age or your genes or where you live or even cigarette smoking. No. The single most important factor is what you eat – your diet.

STRATEGIES FOR PREVENTING 'DEATH BY DIET'

Because we can choose what we eat, we can significantly lower our chances of falling prey to these conditions by our food choices. The great news is that food can also help prevent a long list of other conditions, from Alzheimer's disease to varicose veins, from acne to vertigo. Dr Hippocrates, who lived over 2000 years ago, gave his patients wonderful advice when he told them, 'let your food be your medicine; let your medicine be your food.' Here are four simple ways you can do this.

Eat more plants and less animals

A plant-based diet in today's world is essentially healthier than an animal based one. Five servings of fresh fruit and vegetables per day have now become a standard dietary recommendation by such conservative organisations as the American Medical Association, the American Cancer Society and the American Diabetic Association. Their Jamaican counterparts also echo those sentiments. That's good news! The bad news is that according to recent studies, less than 10 per cent of the US population follows that advice. Jamaica is no different.

I particularly urge the daily consumption of soy-based foods. Soy is virtually a miracle food that protects us from many diseases including the killers mentioned earlier. Look for a soy food high in soy protein isolate to provide you with optimal health benefits. For almost a decade I have used and recommended to my patients and friends a soy protein isolate drink called a shake. A shake can replace a meal and is the easiest and most economical way to have some soy every day.

Take more nutritional supplements

Fortunately, more people are taking nutritional supplements today than ever before. Good news! More and more of my medical colleagues are now recommending supplements to their patients. The American Medical Association has at last changed its mind about supplements. It now recommends that everyone should take daily vitamin and mineral supplements for optimal health. Great news! Bad news – all supplements are not equal. The cheapest brand is not usually best, so choose high quality vitamin and mineral supplements. The usual one-a-day approach is not ideal either. Vitamin and mineral supplements work best when taken with each major meal, three times daily. In addition to the basic vitamins and minerals, I suggest taking a variety of other supplements including antioxidants, refined fish oils and various herbs.

Drink more water

Some experts argue that the most common nutritional deficiency is dehydration – a lack of enough water in the body. Good news – more people have become aware of the importance of water. Bad news – the quality of our drinking water has become awful. Simply boiling your water is not good enough. Even among the expensive bottled waters now commonly available, there are questions about quality. You may need to consider investing in your own water purification system.

Lose the excess fat

Medical science admits that overweight and obesity are the most common indicators of chronic illness in our world. The loss of as little as ten pounds of excess body fat can provide tremendous benefits to your health. Choose a weight-loss program that is effective, nutritionally sound and incorporates the three strategies mentioned above.

> **These four recommendations are provided in a simple dietary program I call 'The Cellular Nutrition Program'. Try it.**

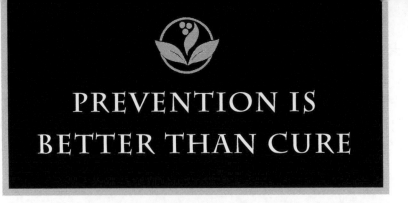

PREVENTION IS BETTER THAN CURE

"An Ounce of Prevention is worth a pound of cure"
– Benjamin Franklyn

No rational person really wants to get sick. That's pretty obvious. Yet so many of us take our health for granted. There is so much we can do to prevent disease. Yet we wait until illness rears its ugly head and then in a panic we desperately try to rescue ourselves. Let me remind you of some of the important reasons why you need to make your health your number one priority.

SIX BIG REASONS NOT TO GET SICK

1. Getting sick makes you feel bad

Being sick prevents you from enjoying life to the fullest, from experiencing what I call wellness. People who eat right, exercise regularly and learn to manage stress while getting adequate rest tend to have a better quality of life than those who don't.

2. Getting sick is expensive

When someone says that they can't afford to follow healthy lifestyle practices, I say you can't afford not to. Sickness is expensive. I have met so many people who have wiped out their life savings in a single illness.

What about health insurance? The term 'health insurance' is a misnomer. It is really 'sickness insurance' and has little to do with health. Although health insurance may sometimes soften the financial burden of disease, how can you insure yourself against the pain, the suffering and loss of time, productivity and happiness that you and your loved ones may face? True health insurance involves spending more of your resources on real health-promoting practices like proper nutrition and exercise.

3. Risk of more sickness

Let's use a simple example. The common cold is the most prevalent illness worldwide. These viral infections of the upper respiratory tract may seem trivial. However, they also leave us vulnerable to other common respiratory complications, including asthma, ear infections, sinusitis and tonsillitis.

Even worse, viral infections can contribute to the development of malignancy. In fact, viruses are considered to be the second most important risk factor for cancer in humans, exceeded only by tobacco use. Examples of common viruses suspected in cancer development include the papilloma virus which can cause cervical cancer, the hepatitis B virus which can cause liver cancer, the Epstein-Barr virus and the herpes virus which can cause blood cancers. Taken together, these viruses are responsible for nearly 20 per cent of cancers worldwide.

4. Exposure to medication

Despite extensive efforts to ensure the safety of prescription drugs, they must be used with great caution. A study in hospitals in the US revealed an extremely high incidence of adverse drug reactions. Even when drugs were taken in the hospital under doctors' directions, there were more than two million adverse reactions each year, many of which contributed to patient deaths. The authors of this study concluded that adverse drug reactions ranked consistently between the fourth and sixth leading causes of death in the US.

Newer drugs are particularly risky, since they have yet to be tested on a large population. Ten per cent of new drugs released over the past 25 years were either withdrawn from the market because of side effects or needed warnings of bad drug reactions. Half of the withdrawals occurred within two years of initial release. The example of the arthritis drug VIOXX® is still fresh in our minds.

Less obvious are the potential dangers of over-the-counter (OTC) drugs. Even though many OTC drugs have been around for a long time, any drug may have unwanted and dangerous effects on some people. Be careful. Use even OTC drugs with caution.

For example, OTC anti-inflammatory drugs can increase the frequency of headaches and raise blood pressure. Doctors have realised that daily use of even mild painkillers, such as Tylenol or Advil, can actually aggravate the headaches that they were designed to treat.

Another US study of a large group of women indicated that those who took aspirin or Tylenol one day or more per month showed a significantly higher risk of developing high blood pressure. The researchers believe that many cases of hypertension in the United States may be due to the use of these medications.

5. Chance of being hospitalised

Hospitals play an important role in our society, and many lives are saved within their walls every year. For example, survival from trauma has increased dramatically because of improved hospital procedures. Nonetheless, hospital environments and procedures are not perfect.

Contrary to the popular belief that hospitals are clean, germ-free environments, many patients actually acquire infections when they are hospitalized. In some intensive care units, as many as 20 per cent of patients develop infections. In the US, 100,000 deaths per year are linked to hospital infections. These infections kill more people each year than car accidents, fires and drowning combined. Fortunately, the hospital infection rates here in Jamaica appear to be much lower.

6. Exposure to medical errors

Overwork, fatigue and chronic staffing shortages among medical workers contribute to treatment errors and problems resulting from incorrectly prescribed or inaccurately filled prescriptions drugs. Death due to medical errors now ranks as the eighth leading cause of death in the US. I have been unable to find any data on this situation in Jamaica.

So if you needed convincing, I hope that you now have six more compelling reasons why an ounce of prevention is worth much more than a pound of cure.

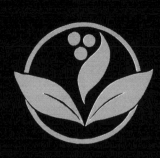

SECTION 2

HEALTHY AGENTS AND PRACTICES

*'The physician should not treat the disease but the
patient who is suffering from it.'*
– Maimonedes, Arabian physician

www.anounceofprevention.org

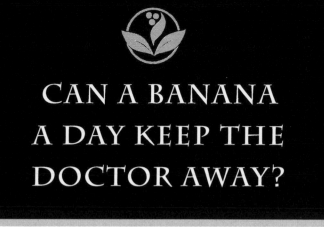

CAN A BANANA
A DAY KEEP THE
DOCTOR AWAY?

Bananas are probably the most popular fruit around the world, with only the orange providing any challenge for that title. Of course, I strongly recommend a high daily intake of fresh fruit and vegetables as a key component of a healthy diet. But, should we be eating lots of bananas, in particular, every day? As with most things, there are two sides to the coin, so let's put the banana under the microscope.

WHAT'S IN A BANANA?

Bananas contain a lot of carbohydrates – three natural sugars (sucrose, fructose and glucose), starch, fibre, some protein, all eight of the essential amino acids particularly the amino acid tryptophan, and hardly any fat.

The banana is a good source of vitamins (especially vitamin B_6) and minerals (particularly potassium, magnesium and iron) as well as water, being a water rich food.

When compared to an apple, a banana has four times the protein, twice the carbohydrate, three times the phosphorus, five times the vitamin A and iron, and twice the other vitamins and minerals, like B_6 and potassium. So it is one of the best value foods around.

Banana's health claims

Bananas have been touted as a useful aid against a wide range of health issues including the following.

- **Depression.** Because of its tryptophan and B vitamin content, bananas have been recommended for depression and mood disorders.

- **Low energy**. Its high sugar content makes bananas a good instant source of energy. Athletes often rely on this fruit for an energy burst.

- **Anaemia.** Because it contains iron, bananas can help to correct iron deficiency anaemia.

- **Premenstrual syndrome.** Because of its B_6 content, banana consumption has been reported to alleviate PMS.

- **High blood pressure.** Because the fruit is extremely high in potassium, yet low in salt, the US Food and Drug Administration has allowed the banana industry to make official claims for the fruit's ability to reduce the risk of blood pressure and stroke.

- **Constipation.** Bananas are high in fibre, and can help people to restore normal bowel action without resorting to laxatives.

- **Stress.** Potassium is a vital mineral, which helps to normalise the heartbeat, sends oxygen to the brain and regulates your body's water balance. When we are stressed, our metabolic rate rises, thereby reducing our potassium levels. These can be rebalanced with the help of a high-potassium banana snack.

- **Skin conditions.** Some alternative medicine therapists have even recommended that the banana can help mosquito bites and warts by rubbing the affected area with the inside of the banana skin. Many people report that this is successful at reducing swelling and irritation of the skin.

A WORD OF CAUTION ABOUT BANANAS

Ripe bananas

The banana contains a lot of sugar: twice the amount found in oranges or apples. It has a rather high glycaemic index. That means that it is a food that significantly raises the blood sugar level. This, in turn, increases the body's production of the hormone insulin.

A number of common health problems can be caused or made worse by high levels of blood sugar and/or high levels of insulin. These include diabetes and pre-diabetes, hypoglycaemia, high blood pressure, obesity, elevated cholesterol or triglyceride levels, gout, heart disease and circulatory disorders.

I therefore recommend that individuals with these conditions or those who are at risk of developing them should consume bananas in moderation. For them, I suggest not more than one banana per day. If you already have blood sugar problems, have only a small banana at a sitting or divide a large banana in two and consume it at separate times during the day.

People on weight loss programs need to be careful about the number of bananas they consume. If you are using protein shakes for meal replacement, add no more than half a banana to your shake.

Green bananas and plantains

Green bananas and plantains have a high starch and low sugar content. As they ripen, the starch is converted into sugar. The riper the fruit, the higher its sugar content. But please note that starch will also elevate the blood sugar level especially when a lot is consumed. This is because excess starch is converted to sugar in the body.

The method of preparation of these two foods is also important to note. Boiled bananas and boiled plantains will lose a significant amount of its vitamins and minerals (like iron) when compared to the raw or baked fruit.

**As Hippocrates said,
'Let your food be your medicine and
your medicine your food.'**

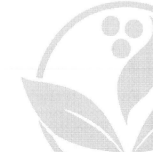

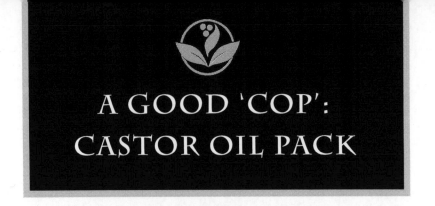

A GOOD 'COP':
CASTOR OIL PACK

The leaves of the trees are for the healing of the nation.
– Revelation 22:2

The oil of the castor bean (*Ricinus communis*) is well known in Jamaica as a cathartic, or strong laxative, but it is no longer very popular because of its unpleasant taste. However, castor oil has been used externally for centuries as a natural therapy. In the famous Edgar Cayce Readings*, castor oil packs (COPs) are strongly recommended to improve elimination of toxins and to enhance the lymphatic circulation. Eventually, in 1980, the active component of castor oil, ricinoleic acid was identified and science began to understand how it works.

HOW COP WORKS

Castor oil appears to have a unique ability to be well absorbed transdermally (through the skin) and to relax smooth muscle. This simple mechanical action has a beneficial influence on all structures with muscular walls, specifically the blood and lymph vessels, the uterus, fallopian tubes, bowels, gall bladder, and even the liver (which is not hollow but is filled with lots of blood vessels).

COPs can be placed on the skin to increase circulation and to promote elimination and healing of the tissues and organs underneath the skin. Good circulation is required for nutrients to be delivered to the cells, and for waste products and inflammatory factors to be removed. COPs are often used to relieve pain, increase lymphatic circulation, reduce inflammation and improve digestion.

USES OF COPs

COPs improve effective circulation through the pelvic area, and are specifically useful in cases of non-cancerous uterine fibroids and ovarian cysts. COPs also relieve ovarian pain and help with healing after a ruptured ovarian cyst. Other conditions that respond to COPs include headaches, liver disorders, constipation, intestinal disorders, gall bladder inflammation and other conditions of toxicity. A COP placed over your liver area helps your liver work more efficiently, including the breaking down of excess oestrogens, the hormones that stimulate the growth of fibroids and some cysts.

MAKING AND USING COPs

A COP is simple to make. I prefer using raw castor oil, though this is becoming scarcer in our local markets. The packs are made by soaking a piece of flannel in castor oil and placing it on the skin. The flannel is covered with a sheet of plastic, and then a hot water bottle is placed over the plastic to heat the pack. With the pack in place, rest for 30 to 60 minutes. Relax using visualisation, meditation, or just sleep. A good time to use COPs is just before bedtime.

To be effective, a COP must be used at least three times a week, although five times a week is better. In cases of a chronic problem, it works best to commit to a six week treatment plan using a COP five times per week, then repeating as necessary. It's wise to consult with a health care provider experienced with this procedure for the best frequency of treatment for your specific health problem.

PRECAUTIONS

Do not use a heated COP for cancerous tumours or ulcers. Don't use it if you are pregnant, breastfeeding or menstruating, and don't apply over broken skin.

As interesting as this all sounds, please remember that there are no quick fixes. You also need to focus on dealing with the root cause of your problem. Diet, nutritional supplements, adequate rest and stress management are an essential part of a holistic approach to any problem. Yes, a COP can be a great tool if you use it wisely.

---

*Edgar Cayce was a famous American spiritual teacher called the Sleeping Prophet because all his teachings and advice was revealed to him while in a trance state.

'A cup a day may keep the doctor away.'

I constantly remind readers that food is powerful medicine. I have extolled the health benefits of foods and spices like coconut, ginger, green tea and soy. Here is another example: cocoa, a traditional Jamaican drink, prevents cancer and heart disease. Harvard University researchers, backed by candy-producer Mars Inc., recently released the results of a ten-year study, revealing that cocoa – rather, the flavanols in cocoa – can substantially reduce the risk of heart disease and cancer.

This interesting study involved a tribe of Indians called the Kuna Indians. Some of these people live in Panama while others live on the San Blas islands just off the coast of Panama. Researchers compared the causes of death in these two groups.

A big difference between both groups was that the Panama Kunas did not consume cocoa regularly, while the San Blas Kunas drank four to five cups of cocoa water per day. The study revealed that the San Blas Kunas, who drank the cocoa water, had a 1,280 per cent lower risk of death from heart disease than the Panama Kunas, and a 630 per cent lower risk of death from cancer.

This is great news for us, as heart disease and cancer are the leading causes of death in Jamaica and the Western world. Cocoa can significantly help in the prevention of cancer and heart disease.

WHAT'S HEALTHY IN COCOA?

Cocoa is rich in substances called flavanols. These are a type of polyphenol which is a chemical that has an antioxidant effect on the body. This means they can destroy free radicals – charged particles, produced by the body, which can damage cells, cause inflammation and trigger diseases like cancer.

Dr Chang Yong Lee and colleagues at Cornell University in New York carried out tests to measure antioxidant levels in tea, red wine and cocoa. A cup of cocoa came out on top in their study suggesting that it was richer in antioxidants than a glass of red wine or a cup of green tea. However, we do not know what quality or strength of tea was used in that study, as high quality green tea has extremely powerful antioxidant properties.

WARNING – COCOA IS NOT CHOCOLATE!

Don't leap to the wrong conclusions and think that chocolate candy and drinks are good medicine. Yes, cocoa is a major ingredient in commercial chocolate products but most chocolate drinks and candy contain large doses of sugar and milk fat to make them sweet and delicious. Eating milk chocolate bars, for example, will not help you prevent cancer or heart disease because adding dairy products and lots of sugar to chocolate effectively cancels out the healthy antioxidants in the cocoa itself. It may taste good, but it's largely useless in preventing cancer and heart disease. Very dark chocolates have more cocoa while white chocolates have no cocoa at all.

A good rule of thumb is to consume chocolate containing a minimum of 70 per cent pure cocoa. Avoid added sugars, artificial sweeteners and milk fat to truly gain the natural anti-cancer benefits of cocoa. The best form in which you can consume cocoa is its most pure form: raw cacao. Cacao is the actual bean that cocoa comes from, and it is one of the richest food sources of flavanols available. It's completely raw, so it hasn't been processed.

The best cocoa is natural cocoa powder or the compressed chocolate sticks sold in the market. Use soy milk instead of cow's milk to make a drink and sweeten with small amounts of dark sugar or stevia. Stevia is a non-caloric vegetable sweetener obtained from the leaves of a Chrysanthemum-like herb native to Paraguay. It is 70 times sweeter than sugar.

The studies also show that drinking cocoa as a hot beverage provides the best health benefits.

VARIETY IS THE SPICE OF LIFE

While consuming cocoa on a regular basis will indeed help you significantly reduce the risk of cancer and heart disease, remember that it is not your only option. A wide variety of foods and beverages contain flavanols: green and black tea, pomegranates, cherries, apples, apricots, blackberries, raspberries, purple grapes, callaloo, kale and other greens. However, for cocoa lovers, the word is out: your favourite food has finally been proven to help prevent cancer and heart disease, the top two causes of death in Jamaica.

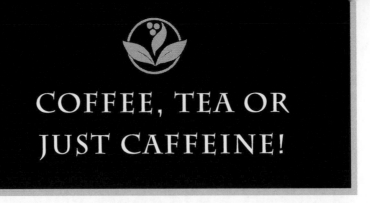

COFFEE, TEA OR JUST CAFFEINE!

For years, I have used and recommended green tea for its incredible health benefits. Tea (primarily black tea) is in fact the most widely consumed beverage on the planet while coffee drinking is still extremely popular around the world. All these beverages have a common constituent – caffeine. What's the truth about caffeine?

WHAT IS CAFFEINE?

Caffeine is known chemically as trimethylxanthine. Medically, caffeine is used to stimulate the heart, to dilate the breathing passages in conditions like asthma and also as a mild diuretic to increase urine production.

Recreationally, it is used to provide a boost of energy or create a feeling of heightened alertness. Caffeine by itself is a brain stimulant and is addictive, as its actions are similar to those of the amphetamine drugs.

Caffeine occurs naturally in many plants, including coffee beans, tea leaves and cocoa nuts. It is important to note however that in these natural food substances, the caffeine exists not in isolation but in combination with hundreds of other active chemicals, which can modulate the actions of caffeine itself.

In her unbounded wisdom, Mother Nature often creates her own checks and balances that we often override by isolating and using one component of a plant. This is what happens when caffeine is added artificially to a wide range of food products including a variety of beverages.

CAFFEINE IN THE DIET

Here are the most common everyday sources of caffeine:

1. **Coffee.** Typical drip-brewed coffee contains 100 mg per six-ounce cup. If you are buying your coffee at a restaurant or fast food outlet or drinking it at home or the office out of a mug, you are consuming it in 12-, 14- or 20-ounce containers. You can calculate the number of milligrams based on your normal serving size.

2. **Tea.** Typical black tea (in regular tea bags) contains 70 mg per six-ounce cup. Green tea contains 30 mg per six-ounce cup.

3. **Others.** Generally, colas (Coca Cola, Pepsi, etc.) contain 50mg per 12-ounce can; cocoa or hot chocolate contains 20mg per six-ounce cup; typical milk chocolate contains 6mg per ounce; Anacin contains 32mg per tablet; No-doze contains 100mg per tablet; Dexatrim contains 200mg per tablet.

BENEFITS OF CAFFEINE

Two hundred milligrams of caffeine has been shown to improve alertness and concentration, and studies have suggested it helps some night-shift workers to maintain concentration, potentially reducing the chances of industrial accidents.

Ingesting 300 mg (equivalent to three six-ounce cups of coffee), 30 minutes before a workout results in up to 30 per cent improvement in endurance with faster times, less exertion, less fatigue and more rapid recovery.

Caffeine is the most active ingredient in many diet pills, as it breaks down fat into fatty acids, which are immediately burned. Conversion of fat to energy is about 30 per cent more efficient when caffeine is consumed prior to exercise. However, this breakdown and burning occurs only when you exercise.

It has been suggested that because caffeine is an antioxidant, it may help prevent the development of some types of cancer.

CAFFEINATED SOFT DRINKS AND CHILDREN

A high caffeine intake is bad for children. It actually dissolves the calcium in young bones. When a group of 13 to 18 year-olds drank an unsweetened caffeinated drink, the calcium output in their urine increased by 25 per cent.

When they drank sugary, caffeinated drinks, their calcium loss was even higher.

Phosphorus, found in most carbonated soft drinks, accelerates bone loss even more. One soda costs a child as much as 120mg of calcium. Furthermore, a soft drink after a workout also depletes children's sodium, chloride, and potassium levels, causing sore muscles and delayed recovery time after exercise.

THE BEST SOURCE OF CAFFEINE

Yes, caffeine is potentially useful, but how much you consume and where you get it from is very important. I believe that the best source of caffeine is green tea. Why?

- Green tea contains much smaller quantities of caffeine than coffee or black tea. It has a powerful energising and fat-burning effect due to other substances it contains.

- Green tea contains potent antioxidants called polyphenols that can prevent cancers like prostate, breast and intestinal cancer. It also has a long list of other health benefits from lowering cholesterol to preventing tooth decay.

- In addition to being energising, green tea also has an anxiety relieving effect. This is due to the presence of a substance called treanine that appears unique to teas.

So when used wisely and in moderation, caffeine can have many health benefits. But I recommend that you get it from green tea.

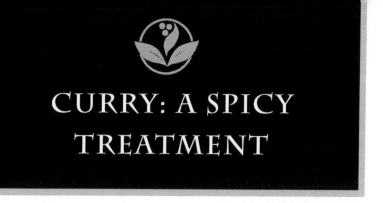

CURRY: A SPICY TREATMENT

If you eat curry dishes regularly, give yourself a pat on the back (or belly). Curry is the signature seasoning in Indian foods and turmeric is the star ingredient in curry mixes. Curcumin is the group of plant pigments that is responsible for turmeric's characteristic canary yellow colour. Researchers have found that curcumin has a wide range of powerful and useful properties. Here's the lowdown on some of the most promising research to date.

MODERN SCIENCE MEETS ANCIENT FOLKLORE

Turmeric (*Curcuma longa*) is a cousin of ginger and is familiar to Indians not only as a spice but also as an important element of folk medicine. In the ancient Indian system of Ayurvedic medicine, turmeric is used to improve overall energy, relieve gas, treat arthritis and improve digestion.

Hundreds of experiments conducted by modern medical researchers around the globe have now demonstrated curcumin's ability to halt or prevent certain types of cancer, stop inflammation, improve cardiovascular health and kill or inhibit the toxic effects of certain microbes including fungi and parasites. As one research team declared, 'Curcumin has been proven to exhibit remarkable anti-cancer, anti-inflammatory and antioxidant properties.'

This hard-working spice even shows promise as a treatment for multiple sclerosis, and may reduce the long-term complications of diabetes. Some researchers have also noted an exciting link between turmeric consumption and a dramatically decreased incidence of Alzheimer's disease, an effect probably related to curcumin's ability to block inflammation. Still other studies have examined curcumin's ability to counteract the effects of toxins in the food, and to protect the eyes from cataracts and uveitis, an inflammation of the eye that may result in glaucoma.

Curcumin for cancer prevention and treatment

Numerous studies published in medical journals detail curcumin's ability to protect against cancer. In addition to its capacity to intervene in the growth of cancer cells and tumours (and to prevent their subsequent spread throughout the body) curcumin has also been shown to increase cancer cells' sensitivity to certain drugs commonly used to combat cancer, rendering chemotherapy more effective in some cases. Researchers at the University of Texas MD Anderson Cancer Center declared, 'Curcumin has enormous potential in the prevention and treatment of cancer.'

Curcumin for lowering cholesterol

Curcumin acts to lower total cholesterol levels. Perhaps even more important, it prevents oxidation of LDL ('bad' cholesterol), which plays a key role in the development of atherosclerosis. Still more intriguing is the finding that curcumin raises HDL (good cholesterol) levels, even as it reduces LDL levels.

Atherosclerosis is a common disorder associated with ageing, diabetes, obesity, and a diet high in saturated fat. It begins gradually, as cholesterol and other lipids deposit on arterial walls and form damaging plaques. As plaques grow, vessel walls may eventually thicken and stiffen, restricting blood flow to target organs and tissues. Atherosclerosis is a major cause of heart disease and may also lead to stroke.

Curcumin for treating malaria

After an absence of half a century, malaria, still a major global health concern, has resurfaced in Jamaica. New, inexpensive and effective anti-malarial agents are urgently needed. Researchers from the Department of Internal Medicine, at the University of Michigan Medical School, have shown that curcumin derived from turmeric inhibits strains of the malaria parasite (*Plasmodium falciparum*) that are resistant to anti-malaria drugs.

Oral administration of curcumin to mice infected with the malaria parasite reduces the level of parasites in the blood by 80 to 90 per cent and enhances their survival significantly.

At the Indian Institute of Science in Bangalore scientists have also shown that the spice protects animals infected with malaria. Two days after they were infected with the malaria parasite, daily doses of curcumin were added to the animals' food for the next five days. Nearly a third were still alive after 20 days, whereas animals not given curcumin had all died by day 13. Thus, curcumin may represent a novel treatment for malarial infection.

SPICE UP YOUR LIFE

Although scientific investigation into the health benefits of curcumin is ongoing, it seems clear that this plant pigment from a humble tuber has powerful healing potential. Adding curcumin to one's diet seems to make exceptionally good sense. Curcumin appears to prevent certain cancers, inhibit heart disease and quell inflammation. It may even offer protection against Alzheimer's disease and malaria.

Because it has been consumed safely by millions of people for literally thousands of years, the choice to supplement one's diet regularly with curcumin would seem to be a no-brainer. One important tip, however: curcumin is poorly absorbed by the gut, but its uptake can be significantly improved by an absorption enhancer called Cell Activator or a black pepper extract called piperine.

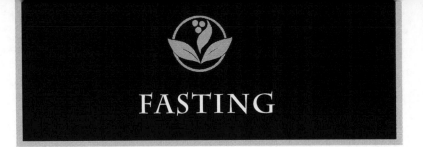

FASTING

'To lengthen thy Life, lessen thy Meals.'
– Benjamin Franklin

Many religious traditions embrace fasting as an important spiritual practice. For Christians, fasting is particularly meaningful during the season of Lent while Muslims traditionally fast during the month of Ramadan. Interestingly, scientific research has demonstrated that fasting might also be very good for your physical health.

In the US, at the National Institute on Ageing, a variety of health benefits have been demonstrated following a 30 per cent reduction in food intake in laboratory animals. These included:

- A significant and lasting reduction in blood sugar levels, blood pressure and heart rate

- An increased ability to handle stress and resist toxins

- Weight loss

- A 30 per cent increase in lifespan

- Reduced risk of cancer

- Enhanced sleep and increased daytime vigour and vitality

- Elevated production of anti-ageing substances, such as growth hormone, DHEA and melatonin

- A general anti-ageing benefit

While a number of practical considerations make it difficult to reproduce this kind of experiment in humans, many experts believe that men and women would get much the same benefits from restricting their overall caloric intake, as long as they ensured that all their nutritional requirements (vitamins, minerals, etc.) were met.

HEALTHY FASTING

Unfortunately, the modern Western diet provides just the opposite: too many calories and too few nutrients. Thankfully, nutritional science has solutions to this dilemma. Here are some tips on how to get not only the spiritual but also the health benefits from fasting this Lent:

1. Select specific fast days. Identify one or more days in the week for your fasting. Try, if possible, to choose days when you will have some time to rest, meditate or pray. Fasting two days per week or on alternate days or on weekends are popular choices. I recommend that prolonged fasting, for more than a few days, should be supervised by a trained health care provider.

It is also important to eat moderately on the days when you are not fasting. Drastically reduce your consumption of meats, fatty and fried foods. Be moderate with the traditional bun and cheese this Easter.

2. Drink liquids instead. I recommend liquid fasts, as they are less strenuous on the system. The liquids consumed can include pure water, soy-based shakes, herbal teas, dilute fruit juices, vegetable juices, coconut water and vegetable broths. Aim at having half an ounce of liquid for each pound of body weight. So, if your weight is 150 lb, you should drink at least 75 ounces of fluid daily while on your liquid fast.

As I have emphasised in the past, breakfast is our most important meal. A wonderful, healthy liquid breakfast would combine a soy-based protein shake along with a cup of herbal green tea. I recommend a specific proprietary blend of soy protein for making the ideal shake. The soy protein shake can also be repeated for the evening meal accompanied by a cup of vegetable broth. You should continue taking your vitamin and mineral supplements while on your liquid fast.

3. Incorporate a cleansing program. Fasting encourages the body to release the toxins and impurities stored in its tissues. Doing a cleansing program while you fast will facilitate the detoxification process while enhancing the health benefits of your fast. I often employ a herbal cleansing program that combines a herbal aloe vera drink along with special fibre tablets called Flora Fiber. Other cleansing modalities like colon irrigation, steam or sauna baths and hydrotherapy are also powerful.

4. **Practise mental hygiene.** Our thoughts and mental activity can also be toxic and unhealthy. Avoid exposing yourself to horror, violence and negative news. Choose carefully what you watch on television and read in the newspapers. Become aware of the thoughts you dwell on and the kind of conversations you have. Be particularly careful of the company you keep. Carry out what a friend of mine refers to as 'mental flossing' and focus on healthy, positive, uplifting thoughts while banishing the negative, unhealthy ones.

Make the commitment to follow a healthy fasting program for Lent. It can make an enormous difference to your health and wellbeing. Even more, it may set the stage for life-changing, long-term health benefits.

A journey of a thousand miles begins with the first step. Make a step towards better health – try fasting.

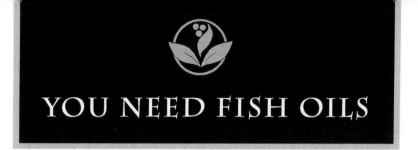

YOU NEED FISH OILS

I have repeatedly encouraged readers to supplement their diet with fish oils. I now return to the subject because medical research continues to discover more and more benefits from this natural supplement.

WHY FISH OILS?

Fish oil is the best dietary source of certain essential fats called omega-3 fatty acids. Omega-3 fatty acids are one of two main groups of key fatty acids – the omega-3 and the omega-6 – that are vital to human life. They are called essential fatty acids (EFAs) because, although the body cannot make them, they are absolutely needed for normal growth and development. These fats must be supplied by the diet. People living in industrialised Western countries eat up to 30 times more omega-6 than omega-3 fatty acids, resulting in a relative deficiency of omega-3 fats.

Too much omega-6 fatty acids creates inflammation that results in allergic and inflammatory disorders and makes the body more prone to heart attacks, strokes, and cancer. Eating diets rich in omega-3 acids and/or taking fish oil supplements can restore the balance between these two types of fatty acids and can possibly reverse these disease processes.

Fish oils for heart disease, cholesterol and stroke

Omega-3 fatty acids are good for the heart. They protect the heart by preventing blood clots and by keeping other harmful fats from injuring the walls of the blood vessels. They not only relax the arteries but also help to prevent thickening of the blood. They can reduce the need for the use of blood thinning medication.

Numerous medical studies have shown that diets rich in omega-3 fatty acids decrease the risk of heart attacks, strokes, and abnormal heartbeats. Clinical trials demonstrate that regular consumption of fish or fish-oil supplements can prevent sudden death due to abnormal heart rhythms. Omega-3 fatty acids are especially useful after menopause in the prevention of heart attacks in women.

In addition, eating omega-3-rich food will result in a lowering of total cholesterol levels, an increase in the concentration of good cholesterol (HDL) and a decrease in the concentration of bad cholesterol (LDL).

Fish oils for high blood pressure

Several studies have shown that eating 200 g of fatty fish or taking 3 to 5 g of high quality fish oil daily will lower blood pressure. Therefore, omega-3 fats can benefit patients who do have high blood pressure while helping to prevent hypertension in those at risk.

Fish oils for babies and children

Omega-3 fatty acids are essential for the normal development of vision and brain function in newborns and children. Human breast milk contains the appropriate amount of omega-3 and omega-6 fats and is best for all babies. This is particularly true if the mother has supplemented her diet with unpolluted fatty fish and/or fish oils. If mother's milk is unavailable, then formulas that provide higher amounts of omega-3 fatty acids are beneficial. Studies have shown that babies given formulas supplemented with essential fatty acids (EFAs) have better vision and score higher in tests, compared to babies on formulas that do not contain additional EFAs.

Fish oils for arthritis

Because omega-3 fatty acids inhibit inflammation and pain, they can help control arthritis symptoms. Significant reduction in the number of tender joints and in morning stiffness, as well as an increase in strength, has been observed in arthritic patients taking fish oil capsules.

Research shows that patients taking fish oil supplements for rheumatoid arthritis require fewer pain medications and may even discontinue their medication completely. Personally, I have patients who have been able to avoid joint replacement surgery by using fish oil and other supplements.

Fish oils for asthma

Taking high doses of omega-3 fatty acids can reduce inflammation of the airways and reduce asthma attacks. According to Donald Rudin, the author of the book entitled *Omega-3 Oils*, allergic disorders, such as asthma, may be triggered by too much omega-6 and too little omega-3 fats in our diet. Fish oil supplements can keep the omega-6 fats in check and decrease the inflammatory reactions associated with asthma.

Fish oils for mental disorders

Research indicates that many common mental disorders such as depression, bipolar disorder (manic-depression), attention-deficit hyperactive disorder (ADHD), anxiety and schizophrenia, may be triggered by deficiencies of omega-3 fatty acids and/or B vitamins. The rates of depression are lower in countries that eat a lot of fish, while the rate steadily rises in countries eating more processed foods and less fresh fish and vegetables containing omega-3 fats.

Supplements containing omega-3 fats have reportedly been effective in children with ADHD precipitated by essential fatty acid deficiencies. Furthermore, a 25 per cent decrease in schizophrenic symptoms was observed in patients taking the omega-3 fatty acids contained in fish oil.

Fish oils for cancer prevention

Omega-3 fatty acids inhibit cancer growth when injected into animals. Flaxseed oil, which is a plant source of omega-3 fatty acids, has been shown to prevent cancer of the breast, colon and prostate. The Mediterranean type diet, high in fish and vegetables, decreases the risk of getting cancer. One study showed that the risk of getting cancer was decreased by over 60 per cent in persons on the Mediterranean diet compared to those on just a low fat and high fibre diet. Omega-3 fats, it seems, strengthen the immune system and inhibit the formation and growth of tumours.

I could go on and on, as in my medical practice I use a specially pure and potent type of fish oil in treating many other conditions ranging from diabetes and hormonal imbalance to high blood sugar, sickle cell anaemia and neuropathy. I just hope that by now you have got the point. Everyone can benefit from supplementing their diet with fish oils.

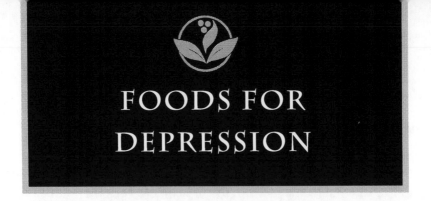

FOODS FOR DEPRESSION

Today we live in a world where more people are mentally unstable. Depression, violence, irrational and anti-social behaviour are escalating in our society. New research published in a medical journal called *Biological Psychiatry* shows that certain foods (which are sadly lacking in our modern diet) are better at treating depression than antidepressant drugs.

This is an exciting finding because it shows yet more scientific evidence of the healing effects of food even on our minds and emotions. Why would one's first choice be antidepressant drugs for treating depression when there are simple, healing foods available that do a better job? This is especially true when considering the potentially dangerous side effects of antidepressant drugs that are now coming to light, including increased risk of suicides, violent behaviour and other similar acts of aggression.

HEALING FOODS

But what healing foods in particular are we talking about in this study? The study found that omega-3 fatty acids and foods high in a compound called uridine were able to reduce the symptoms of depression as well as or better than three popular antidepressant drugs.

Omega-3 fatty acids

Over 60 per cent of the human brain is made of fats. A large portion of the fats in your brain is identical to the omega-3 fats found in fish oils. Your grandmother was right – fish is brain food. Major medical institutions around the world are now using high doses of omega-3 fats to treat depression and other mental illnesses. Even if you are taking antidepressant drugs, fish oils make the drugs more effective and can often replace them. I have, in other chapters, written exhaustively about the many, many other health benefits of fish oils. In my opinion, everyone should take fish oil supplements.

Uridine and molasses

Uridine is chemically described as a nucleotide and is a health enhancing substance found in molasses, walnuts and many other foods. Uridine has a crucial influence on important processes in the human body, particularly in the nervous system where it may act as a nerve growth factor, and seems to improve the energy utilisation in the brain. Research has already documented its use in treating degenerative disorders of the nervous system.

It is especially interesting that molasses is an excellent dietary source of uridine because molasses is produced as a waste product from the sugar industry. When you refine sugar cane juice in order to make refined white sugar, you remove as much as 98 per cent of the nutrition leaving only white, super sweet, highly concentrated refined sugar. Refined white sugar is a potentially toxic food and that is what ultimately gets fed to human beings. The waste product from this is a thick, brown, syrupy liquid – molasses.

Molasses contains most of the nutrition of the sugarcane, including the vitamins, minerals and various compounds such as uridine. It is this molasses that is often used in livestock feed, and yet research is finding that this molasses can help prevent depression. Eating molasses is part of a food strategy that produces effects just as good as antidepressant drugs. Jamaica produces tons of this nutritious and healing food.

The news that these foods can treat depression better than antidepressant drugs may be new to the general public and conventional medicine, but it is old news to those in the fields of holistic nutrition and natural health. We have known for a long time that eating fish, nuts and molasses, and getting good nutrition greatly affects mental health. And we know that most people who suffer from depression are depressed because of a lack of nutrition, whether it is through a lack of nutritionally balanced food or a lack of another natural antidepressant nutrient – natural sunlight.

My experience is that most of the common diseases of modern civilization, like depression, can be treated if not entirely prevented through good nutrition and lifestyle changes.

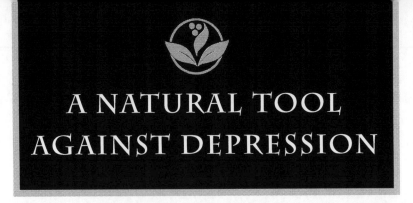

A NATURAL TOOL
AGAINST DEPRESSION

We live in exciting times when many substances that are naturally present in the human body are being discovered and found to have healing properties. Linus Pauling, the double Nobel Prize winner, coined the phrase 'Orthomolecular Medicines' to describe these amazing substances. One such compound is called SAMe, the scientific name for **S-adenosyl-methionine**. This substance is found in every cell in our bodies and, on average, humans produce six to eight grams of SAMe daily. It takes part in several biological reactions in the human body, including balancing brain function, joint cartilage repair, liver detoxification and cell membrane activity. SAMe cannot be obtained directly from the diet, so it is important to eat foods that supply the nutrients that are critical to the synthesis of SAMe in the body. This includes dark green leafy vegetables, whole grains and legumes.

SAMe AND DEPRESSION

Among its many functions, SAMe is essential for the manufacture of certain substances called neurotransmitters that are vital for the healthy functioning of the brain. An imbalance in these substances is now known to be a major factor in depression. Since 1993, over 40 medical trials have been conducted using SAMe in the treatment of depression. The overwhelming consensus of these studies is that SAMe is at least as good as, and probably better than, antidepressant drugs in treating depression. Study after study confirmed that SAMe is not only effective but also remarkably non-toxic with few side effects. It is fast acting and well tolerated even by the elderly or the mentally disturbed.

SAMe – OTHER USES

SAMe has also been found useful in treating osteo-arthritis, liver disease, alcoholism, menopausal symptoms, fibromyalgia, senile dementia and early Alzheimer's disease. This widespread usefulness is related to its effect in improving cellular metabolism and detoxification.

GUIDELINES FOR THE USE OF SAMe

This incredible substance is a non-prescription item that is available in tablet form from health food stores. The customary dosage for SAMe is 400 mg to 1200 mg daily. One can start with 200 mg twice daily and increase up to 400 mg three times daily if necessary. You should not alter or stop any medication prescribed by your doctor without consulting him/her. SAMe is not known to negatively interact with prescription medicines, but often makes antidepressant drugs work better. Benefits are often experienced after a week but optimal results manifest themselves after two weeks of treatment.

It may cause slight nausea in some persons and is best taken with a light carbohydrate snack like fruit. It is not recommended for persons with a particular mental illness called bipolar disorder or manic depression.

Personally, I have been very impressed with the response of my own patients to this safe, natural substance, particularly when used in conjunction with healthy lifestyle practices like proper nutrition, exercise and stress management.

 Give the body the right support and nutrition and it will respond by healing and repairing itself.

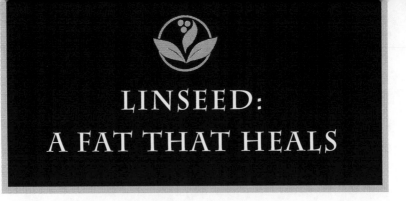

LINSEED:
A FAT THAT HEALS

Not all fats are bad. Some are essential to health but are not manufactured by the body and must be provided in our diet. They are called essential fatty acids (EFAs).

Question: What do depression, fatigue, forgetfulness and a lack of motivation all have in common? What about more serious health conditions like high blood pressure, heart disease, cancer, allergies, other immune disorders, diabetes, arthritis and angina?

Answer: A deficiency or imbalance in the EFAs in our diet.

Scores of health conditions show improvement after supplementing with essential fatty acids. These include Alzheimer's disease, arthritis, cancer, dementia, diabetes, heart disease, lupus, obesity, high blood pressure and psoriasis.

My own clinical experience with the omega-3 fats in fish oil supplements has demonstrated their healing powers. But, there is also a good plant source of essential fats. Flaxseed oil, known in Jamaica as linseed oil, is (after fish oil) probably the richest source of essential fatty acids. Research in Germany has demonstrated the benefits of flax oil as well.

Dr Johanna Budwig was a German biochemist and a leading authority on fats and nutrition. She used these healthy fats to successfully heal patients with cancer, heart diseases, arthritis and other ailments. And this was after conventional medical practitioners had declared these patients incurable. For her work, she received seven nominations for the Nobel Prize.

Her methods were so simple that any housewife could use her techniques with no special training and with good results. In fact, this is exactly what happened in many cases.

THE BUDWIG TREATMENT

The following is not meant to replace medical advice.

Here is Dr Budwig's formula. Get a bottle of linseed oil that is produced with organic flax seeds, cold pressed and protected from oxygen and light. They come in black plastic bottles.

Take a daily mixture of linseed oil and yogurt or cottage cheese at a ratio of one tablespoon of linseed oil to four tablespoons of the yogurt or cottage cheese if you are healthy, and more if you are not well. You can also use a soy protein shake or soy milk. The important thing is to use a high quality protein with the oil and mix them very thoroughly. The linseed oil contains omega-3 oils (which most us are deficient in) which our bodies assimilate better when it is first mixed with a high quality protein. Later, as your body's supply of omega-3 fats is brought up to par, you can reduce the dose.

After taking this oil-protein combination for a day or two, try to get in the sun for at least a half hour or an hour a day and you will feel such a healing effect from the sun that you will be amazed. Dr Budwig used the oil-protein formula as an important element in her methods to cure patients of cancer, heart disease and arthritis.

LINSEED OIL ALSO RICH IN LIGNANS

Linseed is not only rich in essential fatty acids, but is also a rich source of certain phytochemicals called lignans. Linseed contains anywhere from 100 to 800 times the lignans found in other foods. Lignans, like essential fatty acids, can greatly improve our health. They have been found to have antibacterial, anti-fungal and antiviral properties, and recently studies have been focusing on lignans' role in preventing different types of cancer, including breast cancer.

It is estimated that one in eight women will get breast cancer during her lifetime and, unfortunately, many will die from the disease. Research has shown that having too much of the female hormone oestrogen in the body can lead to the development of breast cancer. Studies done on lignans indicate that, in humans, they block the oestrogen receptors from attaching to excess oestrogen, allowing it to be harmlessly eliminated from the body.

A study conducted on 120 women found that those whose breast tissues contained high amounts of omega-3 fatty acids were also the least likely to develop breast cancer. For the women who did get breast cancer, the ones with the higher amounts of omega-3 fats in their breast tissue had the least incidence of spread of the cancer to other organs and tissues.

GENERAL RECOMMENDATIONS ABOUT OILS

- Avoid unhealthy fats, especially saturated animal fats, hydrogenated vegetable oils and trans-fats.

- Use healthy oils like virgin olive oil or virgin coconut oil.

- Include in your diet foods rich in essential fatty acids, like cold water fish, nuts and seeds.

- Supplement with omega-3 fats, especially high quality fish oil and linseed.

- Try Dr Budwig's formula especially if you have any of the health challenges mentioned above.

- For people already supplementing with fish oil capsules, try this alternative. Squeeze the oil from six to eight capsules into a soy protein shake and blend thoroughly. Have a daily sun bath along with your shake.

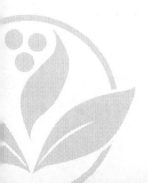

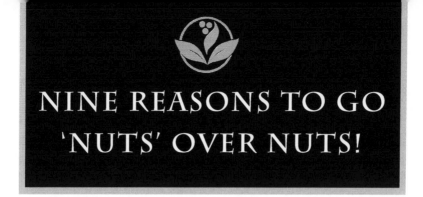

NINE REASONS TO GO 'NUTS' OVER NUTS!

I have often recommended nuts as a healthy addition to our daily diet. Contrary to popular belief, peanuts are not true nuts but legumes, and soy nuts are not true nuts but beans. Nonetheless, they possess many of the same beneficial attributes as most tree nuts.

Here are nine reasons why nuts are great for you.

1. Disease prevention
Medical research confirms that eating one ounce of nuts four to five times weekly can reduce the incidence of heart disease and cancer. In one study, for example, the risk of coronary heart disease was reduced by 35 per cent in those who ate five ounces of nuts per week.

2. Dietary fibre
Nuts can be a good source of fibre, ranging from one gram of fibre provided by one ounce of cashew nuts or pine nuts to three grams in one ounce of hazelnuts, almonds or pecans. Soy nuts may provide even more.

3. Healthy eats
Yes, nuts are high fat foods, but the fats they contain are healthy fats. Nuts are an excellent source of monounsaturated fats, the desirable fat known to lower total cholesterol levels and LDL (bad) cholesterol.

4. Calories
Nuts are a concentrated source of calories, ranging from about 140 calories per ounce for peanuts, and 160 calories per ounce for almonds, pistachios

and cashews to 200 calories per ounce for macadamia nuts. Hence, if nuts are added to your diet and you wish to maintain your current weight, you will need to either increase the calories you burn through exercise or cut back on your calories in other areas of your diet. (If you are a soda drinker, for example, you might consider reducing your intake. A 12-ounce can of soda contains approximately 150 calories.)

5. Magnesium

Nuts are a good source of the mineral magnesium. Almonds and cashews top the list for magnesium. In all the talk about calcium, the great importance of magnesium is often overlooked. Many people are magnesium deficient, particularly those with diabetes or high blood pressure.

6. Selenium

This potent antioxidant is also a mineral with many health benefits including cancer protection. It is exceptionally high in only one nut – the Brazil nut. Just three large Brazil nuts provide approximately 200 micrograms of selenium – the amount recommended for antioxidant protection. One ounce of the other tree nuts, for example, almonds, provides less than five micrograms per ounce.

7. Omega-3 fatty acids

Only two tree nuts – walnuts and pecans – provide the essential fatty acid alpha linolenic acid (ALA). Because the body is incapable of manufacturing this omega-3 fatty acid, it must be obtained from food. Experts suggest that one to two grams be included in the daily diet. One ounce of walnuts contains 2.5 grams of ALA.

8. Protein

Plant-based protein is another offering from the nut family. Macadamias are at the low end, providing two grams per ounce, while soy nuts, pine nuts and pistachios are the powerhouses at seven grams per ounce.

9. Copper

This is another nutrient that can be obtained from nuts. With the exception of macadamia nuts, the majority of tree nuts provide an impressive source of dietary copper, with cashews topping the list.

Anti-Ageing Tip: Include one ounce of nuts five times per week to your diet. Do this by adding whole or chopped nuts to your cereal, salads and desserts. Use as a garnish on vegetables and fruit. Natural peanut butter is a great accompaniment on breads and toast, but did you know that other nut butters are available? Several types, including almond and pecan, are available in many health food stores. Nuts are terrific snacks and make a great addition to many dishes. Have a variety of different nuts for optimal benefit. Experiment and enjoy!

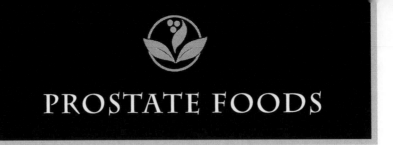

PROSTATE FOODS

Jamaican men have a very high risk of developing prostate cancer. We need to know how to protect ourselves with our most powerful medicine – the food we eat. I have written a lot in the past about the relationship between our food and our risk of developing cancer. I am thrilled to find that modern medical research is now proving my recommendations true. Sadly, hundreds of Jamaican men will die from prostate cancer this year. This does not have to be. The best way to fight it is, of course, through prevention. Here are some prostate cancer prevention foods.

GREEN TEA

Green tea may definitely help prevent prostate cancer in men at risk of developing the disease. Laboratory studies have found that polyphenols, substances in green tea called green tea catechins (GTC), inhibit prostate cancer cell growth in animals. Now researchers have found that these catechins can also prevent the cancer in men.

Italian researchers gave some middle aged male volunteers either tablets of GTC or a placebo (sugar pill) for a year. They found that only three per cent of the men in the group who received GTC developed prostate cancer while 30 per cent of the other men who got a placebo developed the disease.

The green tea compounds killed cancer cells without harming normal cells. Interestingly, the dosage of catechins given to the participants in the study was about that contained in ten cups of green tea – the average amount of green tea consumed daily in China. Chinese men have the lowest rate of prostate cancer in the world.

According to research, drinking green tea may also help prevent the spread of established prostate cancer by stopping the production and spread of new tumour cells. Further, they inhibit the growth of new blood vessels that would nourish the cancer. Please note that the green tea referred to here is not the ordinary 'tea bag' tea that Jamaicans call green tea. I myself use and recommend a patented, potent and tasty form of green tea called Herbal Concentrate Tea.

SOY

There is a food that can reduce your risk of prostate cancer by 70 per cent. It is soy foods: soy milk, soy shakes, soybeans, fermented soy, tofu, and so on. If you consume soy products on a regular basis (one serving a day), *your risk of prostate cancer is slashed by 70 per cent.*

Why is that? There are many phytonutrients in soy products. One of those is called genistein, and it is just one of the many components of soy. It has a powerful anti-tumour effect. This compound blocks an enzyme that destroys vitamin D in cancer cells. So, by blocking this enzyme, vitamin D levels are elevated, and this helps to suppress the growth of cancer tumours. It is important to take both soy and vitamin D (from sunshine) because they work together to create a very positive disease prevention effect.

The fact is that the phytoestrogens (plant hormones) in soy protect the hormone-sensitive prostate gland from cancer. Soy also has high quality proteins and is a great replacement for cancer-promoting meats. Overall, the truth about soy products is wonderful news for people who want to prevent prostate cancer.

My breakfast every day consists of a soy protein-based shake and a cup of Herbal Concentrate green tea. Much research has also been done on other foods that can naturally assist in preventing/treating prostate cancer.

TOMATOES

In a Harvard study involving nearly 48,000 men, researchers found eating tomato sauce a couple of times a week may help prevent prostate cancer. Lycopene (a red pigment) appears to be the active ingredient in tomatoes that is responsible for this effect. Interestingly, lycopene is better absorbed when tomatoes are cooked.

GARLIC, ONIONS AND SCALLIONS

A recent study found that a diet rich in garlic, onions, shallots, leeks and scallions might also cut the risk of prostate cancer. These foods, belonging to the allium group, have previously been found to contain anti-cancer properties. Not surprisingly, China, with the lowest rate of prostate cancer in the world, uses these ingredients as a staple in cooking.

The study surveyed 200 men with prostate cancer and 500 healthy men in Shanghai, China and questioned them on their eating habits. Results published in the *Journal of the National Cancer Institute* were straightforward: men who ate small amounts of onions, garlic, scallions, shallots and leeks each day decreased their risk of prostate cancer by more than 33 per cent.

Additionally, those who ate two grams of garlic per day decreased their risk of prostate cancer by more than 50 per cent, but even eating only one clove cut the risk. Scallions, which lowered the risk of prostate cancer by 70 per cent, were found to be even more beneficial.

Clearly, prevention is the best cure for prostate cancer, and prevention becomes even more possible with the evidence from studies like these.

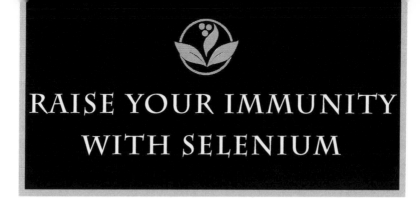

RAISE YOUR IMMUNITY WITH SELENIUM

I have often recommended that readers supplement their diet with the ACES – vitamin A, vitamin C, vitamin E and selenium. I have talked a lot about vitamins A, C, and E. But what about selenium? Selenium is a trace mineral that our bodies use to produce an important enzyme within our cells called glutathione peroxidase, which serves as a natural antioxidant.

Glutathione peroxidase works with vitamin E to protect cell membranes from damage caused by free radicals. Selenium ranks with vitamins A, C and E as a powerful promoter of immunity.

Selenium supplementation has been found to stimulate the activity of white blood cells – a primary component of the immune system. Selenium is also needed to activate thyroid hormones, and it provides protection against a large number of cancers and a broad spectrum of diseases, especially viral infections.

SELENIUM AND HIV/AIDS

The importance of selenium in thwarting viral infections is illustrated by the fact that a number of deadly viruses, such as HIV and Ebola, have emerged from regions in Africa, such as Zaire, which appear to be selenium deficient. On the other hand, despite widespread unprotected promiscuous sexual activity in Senegal, another African country, HIV is spreading very slowly, if at all. The soil in Senegal happens to be rich in selenium.

It has been observed that some people live with an HIV infection for decades before the virus can completely destroy the immune system. Others die within a couple of years of contracting the infection. Strong theoretical evidence suggests that selenium deficiency triggers the progression of HIV infections into full-blown AIDS.

Dr Ethan Taylor, of the University of Georgia, suggested that HIV robs the body of selenium and weakens its immunity. According to Dr Taylor, when the virus uses up all of the selenium in an HIV-infected T cell, it reproduces faster and starts attacking other T cells in its search for more selenium. At some point, the body will not be able to supply enough selenium to quench the thirst of HIV and the signs of full blown AIDS begin to appear.

Ultimately, the entire body's stores of selenium are wiped out by the spreading and selenium-hungry virus. So, selenium availability determines how fast the HIV infection transforms into AIDS. As one expert put it, 'selenium acts as a birth control pill for some viruses like HIV'.

The immune system of the victim of HIV will try desperately to combat the virus by producing large amounts of free radicals to kill the virus and associated bacterial infections. Without glutathione peroxidase and other protective antioxidants, these free radicals become toxic to the immune system itself, and the body becomes even less able to defend itself.

SELENIUM AND OTHER DISEASES

The AIDS pandemic is only one of several ongoing catastrophes involving viruses that encode the selenium-dependent enzyme glutathione peroxidase. Indeed, the world is experiencing simultaneous pandemics caused by the Hepatitis B and C viruses, the Coxsackie B virus along with HIV-1 and HIV-2.

Selenium can also prevent the dangerous mutation of certain types of common viruses, and thus may prevent the creation of new supergerms, like those responsible for bird flu. In many, many ways selenium is essential for healthy immune functioning.

SUPPLEMENTING WITH SELENIUM

In theory, supplemental selenium would do two things. First, it would help keep the person's overall immune system functioning well, and thus prevent viral infections and other immune system problems like cancer. Secondly, supplemental selenium would be very useful in helping the immune system deal with infections that are already present in the body.

Here are my recommendations for supplementation.

1. Eat a selenium rich diet

Good dietary sources of selenium include nuts (Brazil nuts have the highest concentration of selenium of all foods), brewers yeast, fish, oysters, turkey, sunflower seeds, wheat bran, wheat germ, garlic, soybeans and mushrooms. However as modern agriculture uses more and more chemical fertilisers, and with increasing acid rain from environmental pollution, the selenium levels in the soil is lowered. This results in lower selenium levels in our food.

Some countries like New Zealand and Finland are dealing with this problem by enriching the fertiliser used by farmers with selenium. For now, we need to take selenium as a supplement to ensure that we are getting enough in our food.

2. Take selenium supplements

The United States Department of Agriculture states that nutritional supplementation in the range of 50–200 micrograms (mcg) of selenium daily is safe and effective for healthy individuals. The Cellular Nutrition Program that I take and often recommend in combination with immune support supplements will provide well over 100 mcg of selenium daily. The program also provides all the other major antioxidants as well. Remember, antioxidants work best together as a team.

For Hepatitis- or HIV-infected individuals, a higher dose of 400 mcg seems more reasonable, as the disease itself often impairs their absorption of nutrients.

One published clinical study involving actual AIDS patients suggested an even higher daily dose (up to 800 mcg) for a period of several weeks to get their blood levels up, followed by a decrease to 400 mcg, as an effective strategy. Selenium overdosage is very rare and easily reversed.

The selenium story serves to highlight the tremendous importance of good nutrition for optimal health. It shows how devastating a deficiency of one tiny micronutrient can be to the immune system.

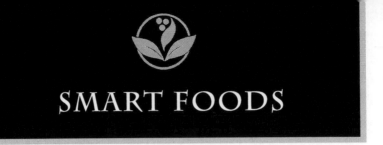

SMART FOODS

Do you ever feel like your brain is in a fog? Is your memory not as sharp as you would like it to be? Well, this doesn't have to be. Certain foods can actually help to boost your brainpower, improve your memory and leave you with better thinking skills. One nutritional specialist, Dr Joseph Mercola, recommends the following foods as they may not only make you appear smarter, they will also contribute to your overall health and wellbeing.

FISH OILS

As the old saying goes, fish is 'brain food'. Unfortunately, fish is more and more contaminated with mercury and dangerous chemicals. What I recommend, however, is fish oil. Packed with beneficial omega-3 fats, fish oil may reduce inflammation in the brain and have a protective effect on our mental function.

Our brains are made up of approximately 60 per cent fat, and most of this fat is the same fat (like DHA) obtained from fish sources. The fats from plant sources like linseed oil have to first be converted by the body into DHA.

When using fish oil or cod liver oil, it is important to obtain a high-quality reputable brand. In my clinical experience with my patients, I have found that certain brands definitely work better than others. For best results, I suggest taking at least twice the dosage recommended on the label.

RAW VEGETABLES

There is little that compares to the nutritional value of organic, raw vegetables. Low levels of folic acid, a nutrient found in green leafy vegetables, have been linked to Alzheimer's disease, and the many antioxidants and phytochemicals in vegetables will help to keep your mind sharp. Dr Mercola suggests that we eat up to one pound of vegetables daily for every 50 pounds of body weight. This can be challenging. The easiest way to achieve this is to regularly drink vegetable juices.

Please note that while I recommend organic vegetables for the most nutritional benefits, if you can't find or afford them, don't use this as an excuse not to eat any vegetables. Eating any vegetables, whether they are organic or not, is much better than not eating any vegetables at all. Just make sure to wash them thoroughly before eating them.

RAW EGGS

Raw whole eggs are an inexpensive and incredible source of high-quality nutrients, especially high-quality protein and fat, that many of us are deficient in. While it may take some getting used to, this is a simple way to improve your mental and overall health. Eating cooked eggs will not have the same effect, and the less you cook the egg, the better it will be nutritionally.

There are several ways to consume raw eggs: a whole egg with the yolk intact swallowed whole; blended in a soy protein shake, or stirred gently into your vegetable juice. Ideally, the eggs should be organic (from healthy free range hens) and as fresh as possible.

FRUIT, ESPECIALLY BERRIES

Berries are among the best fruits on the planet. Not only do they taste great but they are densely packed with a variety of potent phytochemcials that can do wonders to normalise and improve health including direct benefits to the brain. They are also high in fibre and relatively low in sugar, so they won't stimulate severe sugar and insulin swings if eaten in moderation. Imbalances in insulin and sugar are associated with accelerated ageing of the brain.

The best way to eat berries is in their raw, natural state, as heating and freezing can damage antioxidants. However, some antioxidants will remain even after heating or freezing. Different types of berries do contain varying levels of nutrients. Some of the most common and most nutritious berries include blueberries, cherries, cranberries, strawberries and raspberries.

AVOID SUGAR

This is obviously not a food, but more of a food to avoid. If you want to perform at your best, with good memory and intelligence, it is imperative to limit, if not completely avoid, refined sugar.

High-sugar foods will disrupt your body's glucose and insulin levels, which will contribute to disease and brain fog. An easy way to avoid sugar in your diet is to cut out soda and candy, but also watch out for less obvious sources like fruit juice.

So, be smart: eat smart foods.

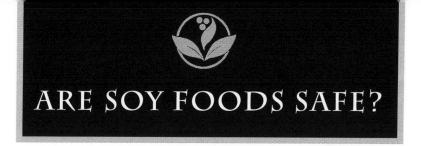

ARE SOY FOODS SAFE?

To my mind, soy is a miracle food. I have been recommending this humble bean to my patients for many years. Scientific research has shown that eating soy protects against heart disease, cancer and osteoporosis while easing the symptoms of menopause. It is also an economical and complete source of protein that can safely replace animal protein in the diet. Yet, from time to time, I have been questioned by people who are concerned about any potential dangers from soy.

Like every good thing, over the years soy has been blamed for all kinds of ills. To my mind, most of these accusations are based on anecdotal reports or shoddy research. The bulk of the evidence confirms the valuable role of soy in preventing disease and supporting health. Let's look at the most common concerns.

SOY AND CANCER

Much of the worry about soy has to do with naturally occurring compounds called phytoestrogens, the most abundant being the isoflavone, genistein. As the name suggests, phytoestrogens have chemical structures similar to that of the hormone oestrogen. This enables them to fit into the body's oestrogen receptor sites, much as a key fits into a lock. Far from causing breast cancer, this ability to bind to oestrogen receptors allows phytoestrogens to block the effects of the much stronger oestrogens that are either produced by the body or come from toxic chemicals like insecticides. This is one mechanism by which soy is thought to protect women against breast cancer.

The majority of research — as well as the experience of Asian populations where soy has been a dietary staple for thousands of years — confirms the protective role of soy. A report published in the May 2001 issue of *Cancer, Epidemiology, Biomarkers & Prevention* provides compelling evidence of the anti-cancer effects of soy foods. This study found that, with an increase in soy intake during adolescence, there was a reduction in the risk of breast cancer. Women with the highest consumption of soy had only half the risk of those with the lowest intake. Other studies have also shown a reduced risk of cancers of the prostate and colon with increasing soy consumption.

SOY AND THE THYROID

Another charge against soy is that it contains 'anti-thyroid agents' that can disturb the function of the thyroid gland. This is largely theoretical. Certain compounds in soy can affect thyroid tissue in test tube studies, but this does not appear to be the case in live human beings.

Population studies show no increased prevalence of thyroid disease in countries with a high intake of soy, and the clinical research has been inconclusive. That debate aside, most researchers agree that consuming soy at the level needed to get its health benefits (about 25 to 40 grams per day) is most unlikely to impair thyroid function. After using soy with hundreds of patients, I have detected no disturbance of thyroid function that I could blame on soy.

However, if you have hypothyroidism, a bit of caution may be in order. Try to keep your soy intake fairly constant and have your thyroid function monitored periodically. Also be aware that taking thyroid medication at the same time as eating soy foods or any foods may decrease the drug's absorption. Take it on an empty stomach.

RECOMMENDATIONS

- Have some soy in your daily diet. Soy is now available in many forms: soymilk, soy cheese, soy nuts, soups, drinks, protein bars, tofu and tempeh. There are also textured vegetable protein products like veggie mince and soy burgers. My favourite way to have high quality soy each day is with a soy protein shake. This is a delicious, nutritious drink that can conveniently replace a meal.

- Select high quality soy products. Many so-called soy products have low levels of the substances that provide the health benefits of soy. Look for the term 'soy protein isolate' and check the protein content on labels as a guide in assessing soy products.

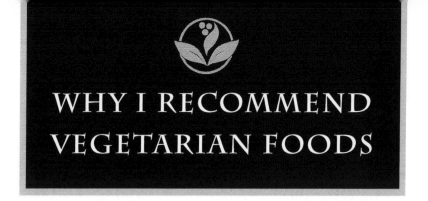

WHY I RECOMMEND VEGETARIAN FOODS

'Nothing will benefit human health and increase chances for survival of life on Earth as much as the evolution to a vegetarian diet.'
– Albert Einstein

For over 15 years I have enjoyed a vegetarian diet and found it to be a powerful way to promote good health. The vegetarian eating pattern is based on a wide variety of foods that are satisfying, delicious and healthy. Vegetarians avoid meat, fish and poultry. Those who include dairy products and eggs in their diets are called lacto-ovo vegetarians. Vegans (pure vegetarians) eat no meat, fish, poultry, eggs or dairy products. Vegetarian diets significantly reduce the risk of a broad range of health concerns.

An American-based medical organisation called Physicians for Responsible Medicine have published the results of their research on the health benefits of a vegetarian diet. Here are their findings.

A HEALTHY HEART

Vegetarians have much lower cholesterol levels than meat eaters, and heart disease is uncommon in vegetarians. The reasons are not hard to find. Vegetarian meals are typically low in saturated fat and usually contain little or no cholesterol, since cholesterol is found only in animal products. Vegans, therefore, consume a cholesterol-free diet.

The type of protein in a vegetarian diet may be another important advantage. Many studies show that replacing animal protein with plant protein lowers blood cholesterol levels, even if the amount of fat in the diet stays the same. Those studies show that a low-fat, vegetarian diet has a clear advantage over other diets.

LOW BLOOD PRESSURE

Studies, dating back to the early 1920s, show that vegetarians have lower blood pressure than non-vegetarians do. In fact, some studies have shown that adding meat to a vegetarian diet raises blood pressure levels rapidly and significantly. When patients with high blood pressure begin a vegetarian diet, many are able to eliminate their need for medication.

DIABETES CONTROL

The latest studies on diabetes show that a diet high in plant protein and complex carbohydrates (soy is a great source) and low in fat is the best dietary prescription for controlling diabetes. Since diabetics are at high risk for heart disease, avoiding fat and cholesterol is important, and a vegetarian diet is ideal. Even insulin-dependent diabetics can help to reduce their insulin needs with a plant-based diet.

CANCER PREVENTION

A vegetarian diet helps prevent cancer. Studies of vegetarians show that death rates from cancer are only about one-half to three-quarters of those of the general population. Breast cancer rates are dramatically lower in countries where diets are typically plant-based. When people from those countries adopt a Western, meat-based diet, their rates of breast cancer soar.

Vegetarians also have significantly less colon cancer than meat eaters. Meat consumption is more closely associated with colon cancer than any other dietary factor.

Why do vegetarian diets help protect against cancer? First, they are lower in fat and higher in fibre than meat-based diets. But other factors are important, too. For example, vegetarians usually consume more antioxidants, like vitamin C and beta-carotene. This might help to explain why they have less lung cancer.

One study has shown that the sugars in dairy products may raise the risk of ovarian cancer in some women. Many of the other anti-cancer aspects of a vegetarian diet are yet to be fully understood.

OSTEOPOROSIS PREVENTION

Vegetarians are less likely to form either kidney stones or gallstones. In addition, vegetarians may also be at lower risk for osteoporosis. A high intake of animal protein encourages the loss of calcium from the bones. Replacing animal products with plant foods reduces the amount of calcium lost. People who live in countries where the diet is plant-based have little osteoporosis, even when calcium intake is low.

SPECIAL CONSIDERATIONS

It is easy to plan a balanced vegetarian diet. Grains, beans and vegetables are rich in protein and iron. Green leafy vegetables, beans, lentils, nuts, and dried fruits are excellent sources of vitamins and minerals.

Vitamin B_{12} is plentiful in fortified foods. Some sources are soy products, commercial breakfast cereals and nutritional yeast. Although vitamin B_{12} deficiency is uncommon, strict vegetarians should be sure to include a source of this vitamin in their diet.

For optimal nutrition, the American Medical Association now recommends that everyone take daily supplements. I use an excellent Cellular Nutritional Program for myself and for my patients.

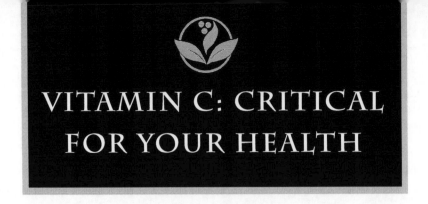

VITAMIN C: CRITICAL FOR YOUR HEALTH

*'There are more than ten thousand published scientific papers that
make it quite clear that there is not one body process and not one
disease that is not influenced directly or indirectly by vitamin C.'*
– Dr Emanuel Cheraskin et al.

Ascorbic acid, popularly known as vitamin C, is perhaps the most impor-tant of the vitamins. Unfortunately, this vitamin is very poorly understood, even by many health professionals. The fact is that vitamin C is essential for life and health. Without it, we would die. Almost all animals man-ufacture their own vitamin C in their bodies and can vary how much they produce. If an animal gets sick or suffers an injury, it automatically increases its production of vitamin C as much as tenfold. Man is the rare exception. We must get our supply of this essential substance from our diet or from supplements.

WHO SHOULD TAKE VITAMIN C?

Everyone should! Our planet Earth is polluted and our food supply is con-taminated. Also, our methods of farming, storing and cooking significantly deplete the levels of vitamin C in the foods we eat. For example, the vitamin C content of broccoli today is 30 per cent less than broccoli grown 30 years ago. If you cut up a cucumber and leave it on your kitchen table for only half an hour, it will lose 20 per cent of its vitamin C content.

We all need more vitamin C than we currently get from our diet. Why is this fact not widely publicized? I suspect that it is because vitamin C is a nat-ural substance and cannot be patented. There is, therefore, no real financial incentive for the pharmaceutical companies or the medical profession to promote this extraordinary nutrient. How sad!

HOW MUCH VITAMIN C DO WE NEED?

The answer is dependent on your state of health. The sicker you are, or the more unhealthy your lifestyle, the more is needed. There is also a significant difference between the amount that is needed to prevent scurvy (the disease caused by severe vitamin C deficiency) and the amount that is needed for optimal health. The recommended daily allowance (RDA) is less than 100 milligrams. However, if you only take the RDA, for example, and smoke more than four cigarettes a day, you will be vitamin C deficient.

Most, if not all of the common illnesses, including stress disorders, allergies, viral infections, traumas, malignancy, stroke and heart attacks, to name a few, dramatically increase the body's need for vitamin C.

HOW TO TAKE VITAMIN C

Eat foods that are rich in vitamin C. Fresh fruits and vegetables are the best sources. These foods, in addition to providing vitamin C, also provide other nutrients and vitamins. However, to get even 1,000 milligrams of vitamin C from food alone you would have to eat the equivalent of 30 oranges per day. This is hardly possible. Supplementation is therefore necessary.

Anyone interested in optimal wellness and/or healing needs to take additional amounts of vitamin C. This can be in the form of tablets, dissolvable tablets or as a powder or crystals. In certain situations involving illness, fatigue, allergies, cancer and other problems with the immune system, it is recommended that vitamin C be given by a doctor in even larger amounts via an intravenous drip.

Vitamin C is best taken in divided doses throughout the day. There is a simple way to decide how much is optimal for you. Start at 1000 mg three times per day and increase by an additional 1000 mg each day. If you exceed your optimal dose of vitamin C, you may experience diarrhoea. This is a sign that your body's tissues are fully saturated with the vitamin. Simply cut back on the amount to a level that your stools are no longer loose, and this is your ideal optimal dosage.

DOES VITAMIN C HAVE ANY SIDE EFFECTS?

This is an extremely safe and natural substance that is essential for the effective functioning of every cell in the body. There is only one undisputed side effect of vitamin C – diarrhoea. The dose at which this occurs is called the *bowel tolerance level* and, as explained earlier, can be used as a guide in determining your appropriate dose of the vitamin. A single large oral dose of vitamin C can act in the same way as a handful of prunes and provides a useful alternative for over the counter remedies for constipation

Vitamin C is water-soluble and any excess is easily excreted in the urine. Even that which is in the urine is not wasted, as it helps to protect the kidneys and bladder from infections and cancer.

There is no truth or medical evidence for the rumour that vitamin C causes kidney stones. In fact, it may very well help to prevent them! Since vitamin C is acidic, persons with stomach acidity will benefit by taking a buffered form of this vitamin (for example, magnesium ascorbate).

Remember that your ideal dosage may vary from time to time depending on your current health status.

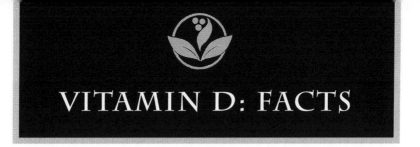

VITAMIN D: FACTS

Vitamin D prevents osteoporosis, depression, prostate cancer and breast cancer, and even affects diabetes and obesity. Vitamin D is perhaps the single most underrated nutrient in the world, probably because it is free: your body makes it when sunlight touches your skin. Drug companies can't sell you sunlight, so there's no promotion of its health benefits. The truth is, most people don't know the real story of vitamin D and health.

At a medical conference, I heard a presentation by an American dermatologist, Dr Michael Holick. His message was simple: sensible exposure to natural sunlight is the simplest, easiest and most important strategy for improving your health with vitamin D. I urge you to read Dr Holick's book, *The UV Advantage*, to get the full story on natural sunlight.

Here is a summary of an interview between writer Mike Adams and Dr Michael Holick.

1. Vitamin D is produced by your skin in response to exposure to ultraviolet radiation from natural sunlight. It is nearly impossible to get adequate amounts of vitamin D from your diet. Sunlight exposure is the only reliable way to generate vitamin D in your own body.

2. A person would have to drink ten large glasses of vitamin D fortified milk each day just to get minimum levels of vitamin D into their diet.

3. The further you live from the equator, the longer the exposure to the sun you need in order to generate vitamin D. Canada, the UK and most US states are far from the equator.

4. People with dark skin pigmentation may need 20 to 30 times as much exposure to sunlight as fair-skinned people to generate the same amount of vitamin D. That's why prostate cancer is an epidemic among black men – it's a simple, but widespread, sunlight deficiency.

5. Sufficient levels of vitamin D are crucial for calcium absorption in your intestines. Without sufficient vitamin D, your body cannot absorb calcium, rendering calcium supplements useless.

6. Chronic vitamin D deficiency cannot be reversed overnight: it takes months of vitamin D supplementation and sunlight exposure to rebuild the body's bones and nervous system. The healing rays of natural sunlight (that generate vitamin D in your skin) cannot penetrate glass. So you don't generate vitamin D when sitting in your car or home.

7. Even weak sunscreens (SPF 8) block your body's ability to generate vitamin D by 95 per cent. This is how sunscreen products actually cause disease – by creating a critical vitamin deficiency in the body. The sunscreen industry doesn't want you to know that your body actually needs sunlight exposure because that realisation would mean lower sales of sunscreen products.

8. It is impossible to generate too much vitamin D in your body from sunlight exposure: your body will self-regulate and only generate what it needs. If it hurts to press firmly on your sternum (breast bone), you may be suffering from chronic vitamin D deficiency right now.

9. Vitamin D is activated in your body by your kidneys and liver before it can be used. Therefore, having kidney disease or liver damage can greatly impair your body's ability to activate circulating vitamin D.

10. Even though vitamin D is one of the most powerful healing agents, your body makes it absolutely free. No prescription required.

What about sunburn, skin damage and skin cancer? It turns out that antioxidants greatly boost your body's ability to handle sunlight without damage or burning. So take enough vitamins A, C and E and eat lots of fresh fruit and vegetables. I take a large dose of vitamin C if I will be exposed to the sun for a long time and I never get sunburn anymore.

'8 glasses a day keep the doctor (and the fat) away.'

According to *Webster's New Lexicon Dictionary*, water (H_2O) is the transparent, colourless liquid which falls from the sky as rain, issues from the ground in springs and composes three quarters of the earth's surface in the form of seas, rivers, lakes, and so on.

Water is probably the single most important catalyst in losing weight and keeping it off. One of the things we take most for granted, water plays a very important role in permanent weight loss. It aids in suppressing the appetite naturally and metabolising stored fat.

Studies show that a decrease in water intake causes fat deposits to increase, whereas an increase in water intake can actually reduce fat deposits. The kidneys do not function properly without enough water. When this occurs, some of the load is passed on to the liver. The liver works to metabolise stored fat into usable energy for the body. If the liver aids the kidneys, it cannot function effectively. Consequently, the liver will metabolise less fat, and the fat will remain stored in the body causing weight loss to cease.

Many people whose bodies retain water drink less water, hoping to eliminate the problem. The body sees the action as a threat to its survival, so it holds on to every drop. Water is then stored in spaces outside the body's cell. This causes swollen feet, hands and legs. Diuretics offer only temporary relief. The best way to overcome excess water retention is to give the body what it needs – plenty of water. Only then can stored water be released.

Overweight people need more water than thin people do, because they have a larger metabolic load. Water also helps to maintain proper muscle tone by giving muscles their natural ability to contract and by preventing dehydration. It helps prevent sagging skin that usually appears following weight loss. Shrinking cells are plumped by water. The complexion then appears clean, healthy and radiant.

Water also flushes waste from the body and thus eliminates constipation. The function of the endocrine glands improves, thus the entire system functions more effectively. Water not only accomplishes all the things listed above, it works with fibre to create a satisfied feeling and helps subdue hunger pains.

HOW MUCH WATER?

That depends on several factors, including your weight. It is recommended that for each pound of body weight you drink half an ounce of water per day. Thus a 200 pound man should aim to consume 100 ounces of water daily. If you are exercising, sweating a lot or are in a hot climate then you need to drink even more. As a general principle, aim to drink eight eight-ounce glasses of water per day, if you live in the tropics.

Here is a simple scheme of how to drink eight glasses of water each day:

1. On rising in the morning, immediately drink one glass of water.

2. Drink one glass half an hour before breakfast, lunch and dinner.

3. Drink one glass half an hour after breakfast, lunch and dinner.

4. Drink one glass before bedtime.

That will get you to eight glasses. In addition, try eating lots of water rich foods such as fruits and vegetables, and liquid foods like shakes and soups.

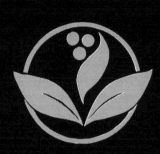

SECTION 3

GENERAL PROBLEMS

*"The doctor of the future will give no medicine,
but will interest his [or her] patients in the care of
the human frame, in a [proper] diet and in the cause
and the prevention of disease."*

– Thomas A. Edison (1846–1931)

www.anounceofprevention.org

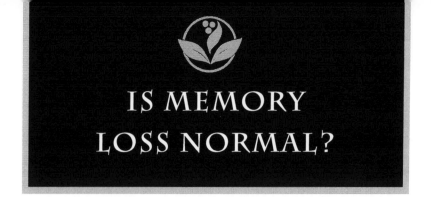

IS MEMORY LOSS NORMAL?

Today we will look at the business of memory and memory loss. The human brain is a very complex organ with the capacity to store vast amounts of information. The experts say that every single event in our lives, from earliest infancy up to the present, is all recorded and stored in our brain's memory banks.

HOW DOES THE BRAIN STORE INFORMATION?

Information is stored in different parts of your brain as memory. Information stored in the **short-term memory** may include the name of a person you met moments ago while information stored in the **mid-term memory** may include what you ate for breakfast. In the **long-term memory** is stored your memories of years ago, such as memories of childhood.

THE AGEING BRAIN AND MEMORY LOSS

Starting in your twenties, you begin to lose a few brain cells at a time on a daily basis. Your brain cells communicate with each other via chemicals called neurotransmitters, and your body also starts to make less of these chemicals in your brain cells as you age. The older you are, the more these changes can affect your memory.

Ageing may affect memory by changing the way your brain stores information and by making it harder to recall stored information. Your long-term memories are usually less affected by ageing than your short-term memory. You may forget names of people you've met recently and remember incidents from your childhood.

Other causes of memory problems

Many things other than ageing can cause memory problems. These include:

- depression
- other illnesses
- dementia (severe problems with memory and thinking, such as Alzheimer's disease)
- side effects of drugs
- hormone imbalance
- stroke
- head injury
- alcoholism.

Alzheimer's disease: A special memory disorder

Alzheimer's disease starts by changing your recent memory. At first, a person with Alzheimer's disease will remember even small details of his or her distant past but not be able to remember recent events or conversations. Over time, the disease affects all parts of the memory.

Alzheimer's disease isn't a normal part of ageing, but it does occur with increasing frequency with ageing. Only 10 per cent of people over age 65 have Alzheimer's disease, but this number increases to nearly 50 per cent of people over age 85.

HOW TO TELL IF MEMORY PROBLEMS ARE SERIOUS

A memory problem is serious when it affects your daily living. If you only sometimes forget names, you're probably okay. But you may have a more serious problem if you have trouble remembering how to do things you've done many times before, like getting to a place you have often been to, or doing things that involve several steps, like following a recipe.

Here are some more memory problems that aren't part of normal ageing.

- Forgetting things much more often than you used to
- Trouble learning new things

- Repeating phrases or stories in the same conversation
- Trouble making choices or handling money
- Not being able to keep track of what happens each day.

Another difference between normal memory loss and dementia is that normal memory loss doesn't get much worse over time. Dementia, however, gets much worse over several months to several years. It may be hard to figure out on your own if you have a serious problem. Talk to your family doctor about any concerns you have. Your doctor may be able to help you if your memory problems are caused by any medication you're taking or by depression.

LIFESTYLE HABITS TO ENHANCE MEMORY

Nourish your brain

Good nutrition is essential to brain health. Recent research has shown that the same dietary factors that promote the development of diabetes can also put you at risk for developing Alzheimer's disease. I recommend the use of the Cellular Nutrition Program to supplement a balanced diet rich in fresh fruit and vegetables along with adequate healthy proteins. What you eat affects everything.

I also recommend taking the following supplements:

- Fish oils (omega-3 fatty acids) in large quantities. The brain is a fatty organ, mostly essential fatty acids.
- B complex and B_{12} vitamins which are essential for a healthy brain
- Antioxidants – Vitamins A, C and E and selenium (the ACES)
- Ginkgo Biloba, which is shown to improve blood flow to the brain
- Guarana, a Brazilian herb available as a tea or tablet called NRG
- Phosphatidylserine, a brain nutrient often called PS
- Alpha Lipoic Acid, another powerful antioxidant
- Ginseng, a tonic herb for the nervous system
- DHEA and Pregnenalone, natural hormones found in the brain.

EXERCISE YOUR BODY, STIMULATE YOUR MIND, AND BE POSITIVE

In one of the best-known studies on ageing, researchers identified healthy people between the ages of 70 and 80 with the highest mental abilities in their age group. They tracked these high performers for years to determine why they retained high mental functioning. Three factors distinguished these people from others:

- **They exercised:** They were more consistently physically active than the others. For example, they took daily walks and other forms of exercise.

- **They remained mentally active:** These were the people who, rather than parking themselves in front of the TV, did the crossword puzzle every morning, browsed the library shelves regularly for new and interesting books, dabbled in hobbies and crafts, or played bridge three times per week.

- **They remained positive:** They had a personality quality some have termed 'self-efficacy'. They met challenges with the confidence and desire to solve them, rather than being victims of misfortune.

Develop your brain

An important guiding principle is the 'use it or lose it' principle. In a study reported in the January 2004 publication of the journal *Nature,* 23 healthy people, with an average age of 22, learned how to juggle. After three months, MRI scans showed enlargement of the gray matter in their brains. The gray matter is the part of the brain responsible for higher mental functions. The scans revealed that either the existing cells had grown larger, with more connections, or the sheer number of brain cells had increased. When the study participants stopped juggling, their brains shrank again. This doesn't mean we should all juggle our way to mental vitality. But it does strongly suggest that mental exercise has real and positive effects on brain function.

So, be reassured that there are many things that you can do to preserve your memory and maintain good brain function.

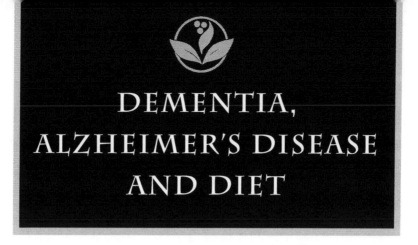

DEMENTIA, ALZHEIMER'S DISEASE AND DIET

*'If I'd known I was going to live so long,
I'd have taken better care of myself.'*
– Leon Eldred

One of the greatest fears that people suffer as they get older is the fear of losing their mental function. But did you know that what you eat could affect your brain function? Let's begin by looking at some definitions.

DEMENTIA

This is the usually progressive deterioration of mental function, such as memory, that can occur while other brain functions, such as those controlling movement and the senses, are retained.

SENILE DEMENTIA

This is a form of brain disorder marked by progressive and irreversible memory loss and disorientation known to affect people after the age of about 65 years.

ALZHEIMER'S DISEASE

This is a form of dementia. Although all patients with Alzheimer's disease have dementia, not all dementia patients have Alzheimer's disease. Alzheimer's disease is the most common neurodegenerative disorder and the major cause of senile dementia.

The Alzheimer's Association defines Alzheimer's disease as an irreversible, progressive brain disease that slowly destroys memory and thinking skills, eventually even the ability to carry out the simplest tasks, ending inevitably in death.

Alzheimer's Disease was named after a German physician, Alois Alzheimer, who first identified the condition in 1906 when he performed an autopsy on the brain of a woman who'd been suffering severe memory loss and confusion for years.

The cause of Alzheimer's disease

Abnormal deposits of specific proteins inside the brain disrupt normal brain function and cause the problems typically associated with Alzheimer's disease. Eventually, as the deposits spread throughout the brain, brain tissue starts dying, leading to further impairment. The resulting brain shrinkage can be seen in CT scans and MRIs. Current research is focused on trying to determine what causes these deposits and is looking for ways to prevent or reverse them before they cause permanent brain damage.

Although there does seem to be a genetic predisposition for the disease, other factors including diet significantly influence whether or not an individual develops Alzheimer's disease.

DIET AND DEMENTIA

Research suggests that your diet may be a very important factor in preventing dementia. Here are some guidelines for you to follow.

Lower your fat intake

A high dietary fat intake (especially animal fat) is associated with an increased risk of developing dementia. The prevalence of Alzheimer's disease is lower in countries where dietary fat and caloric content is lower. A high intake of linoleic acid (a polyunsaturated fatty acid), found in margarine, butter and other dairy products, is positively associated with impairment of mental function.

Be cautious with alcohol

While heavy alcohol consumption is definitely associated with accelerated brain damage, moderate consumption (one to two glasses per day) of red wine is associated with a decreased incidence of dementia. This may be related to the antioxidant effects of the flavinoids in red wine.

Supplement with fish oils

A new Canadian study suggests a diet rich in omega-3 fatty acids, found in fish such as salmon and sardines, and in fish-oil capsules, can help keep Alzheimer's disease at bay. The research provides the strongest evidence so far that a deficiency in a specific dietary component can have a direct impact on a person's risk of developing the devastating disease.

Frederic Calon, a researcher at the Laval University Medical Centre in Quebec City declared, 'What the public needs to take from this is that diet matters to your brain. If you have a diet that is poor in omega-3s, that will accelerate the process of Alzheimer's, especially if you're genetically predisposed.'

Eat more fruits and vegetables

According to a study done at Boston University and Tufts University, people with high blood levels of a dietary by-product, called homocysteine, have twice the average risk of developing Alzheimer's disease. Homocysteine is an amino acid whose levels can rise when people eat too few fruits or leafy vegetables.

Fruits and vegetables are essential in providing B vitamins to the human body. I recommend that adults have seven or more servings of vegetables and fruit daily.

Take dietary supplements

I recommend a wide range of supplements for optimal brain function:

- **B complex vitamins:** These are vital for a healthy nervous system and are needed in greater quantities when you are under stress. They will also lower elevated homocysteine levels. Special attention must be paid to maintaining optimal levels of vitamin B_{12} in your blood.

- **The antioxidants ACES:** Vitamins A, C and E, and selenium. These protect the brain cells and their delicate membranes from damage from free radicals – chemicals in the body that can have toxic effects.

- **Brain nutrients:** Phosphatidyl serene, lecithin, choline and Coenzyme Q10. The brain nutrients (along with fish oils) supply the building materials for brain cells.

- **Herbs:** Ginkgo biloba increases blood flow to the brain while ginseng increases mental energy.

- **Hormones:** Dehydroepiandrosterone (DHEA), melatonin, pregnenelone and progesterone. These hormones essentially slow down the ageing process in the brain.

Avoid aluminium

Aluminium is the third most abundant element in the Earth's crust. In addition to the many dietary sources of aluminium, such as cheese, beer, antacid tablets, some teas, toothpaste, infant formula, aluminium cookware, drinking water and pharmaceutical products, people are also exposed to aluminium by applying deodorants to the skin and by the inhalation of aluminium dust.

While the cause of Alzheimer's disease is still for the most part unknown, several experts have suggested that aluminium plays a role in the disease. There is still major controversy about this issue, but for now I definitely recommend that we seek to minimize our exposure to aluminium.

The bottom line is that there is a great deal we can do to avoid this clear and present danger.

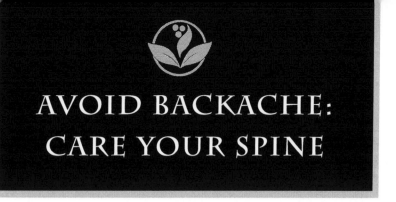

AVOID BACKACHE: CARE YOUR SPINE

Backache is a common complaint and is second only to the common cold as the commonest cause for absence from work. Millions of man/woman hours of production are lost from work every year because of backache, not to mention the suffering of and expense to the individuals who fall victim to this problem. Almost half of all working adults complain of backache every year.

Your backbone (spine) is extremely important to your health. The entire body is under the control of the nerves that originate in the spinal cord. Any disturbance in the alignment of the spine can cause pressure, irritation or inflammation to these nerves and result in a wide range of disturbances and malfunctions in various parts of the body. Backache is often a symptom of a spine that is out of alignment.

A NEW THERAPY FOR A HEALTHY BODY AND SPINE

According to ancient Chinese medicine, the spine must be properly aligned so that there is no pressure on the spinal cord. This allows the flow of *chi* (the body's vital energy) to be undisturbed, and balance to be maintained. If our spine is out of alignment, our health starts failing. In oriental science, doctors treat the whole body instead of trying to fix just one malfunction or symptom. Everything is part of a much bigger system which, if strong, can either prevent illness or heal an existing problem with very little help.

I have been using a new technology called **Livelong** based on chiropractic principles combined with those of traditional Chinese medicine. By lying on this **Livelong** device, the individual receives a therapeutic combination of the following, which helps to keep the spine healthy and alleviate backache:

1. Spinal massage
2. Chiropractic principles
3. Acupressure/Moxibustion
4. Far infrared light/Heat/Jade

Spinal massage

Spinal massage relaxes muscles and tendons around the spine, relieving pressure from the spinal cord, unblocking nerves, and adjusting the spine. The spinal massage also prepares our backs for the other components of the whole treatment.

Chiropractic principles

Have you ever been to a chiropractor? Chiropractic physicians are particularly trained to deal with problems related to misalignment of the backbone. Chiropractic treatment can be extremely effective in correcting backpain and other problems related to the spine. Unfortunately, there are only a few chiropractors currently practising in Jamaica. Along with the benefits of spinal massage, the device called **Livelong** helps to create correct alignment using chiropractic principles.

Acupressure and moxibustion

Acupressure and moxibustion are variations of acupuncture in which specific points on the back are stimulated with pressure and heat, respectively, instead of needles. These techniques unblock what in oriental science are called meridians, or the 12 energy channels along which *chi* flows. Acupuncture is probably one of the most popular techniques used in oriental medicine and, although **Livelong** uses no needles, it causes exactly the same effect, with different tools.

According to oriental medicine, illness starts when the *chi* flow is disturbed. To maintain or restore *chi* flow, different techniques can be applied, such as acupuncture, acupressure, and moxibustion.

Far infrared light/heat

Going back to the principles of oriental medicine, proper blood circulation and clean blood are essential for our wellbeing. **Livelong** uses jade projectors and carbon panels which produce heat and far infrared light.

Both heat and light are essential in the healing process and in the detoxifying process. Heat and far infrared light help the body to slowly clean the toxins from our system. They also help the body to generate blood from the bone marrow, which is important, especially for those whose immune systems are weak.

Along with heat, far infrared light penetrates deep into the body, reducing swelling and inflammation and promoting healing, in a safe and non-invasive way. Jade is a semi-precious stone which, for ages, has been used in oriental medicine to help stimulate *chi*. Jade is incorporated in the **Livelong** device because of its ability to hold and transmit heat and far infrared light into our bodies.

Livelong is not just a temporary measure to treat, control or diminish symptoms of a particular condition. It does and will help the body to start curing or improving our problems, but it is also about maintenance and prevention! Daily adjustments of the spine, detoxifying, maintaining blood and *chi* circulation result in our bodies being strong and able to fight and prevent diseases.

The world is changing. This change is making us struggle even harder to maintain a healthy life. Through extensive scientific research and development, the **Livelong** technology has successfully integrated the traditional principles of Eastern and Western medicine and it is now available right here in Jamaica.

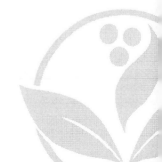

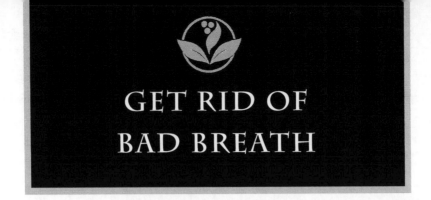

GET RID OF
BAD BREATH

THE PROBLEM

Bad breath is a common social problem that can also be an important indicator of poor health. The medical term for bad breath is halitosis, and according to the National Institute of Dental Research in the US, over 65 million Americans suffer from it. In my experience, Jamaicans have their fair share of halitosis too. In Israel, people have actually been sued and even divorced for bad breath!

THE CAUSE

Many factors can contribute to bad breath: dental problems, diabetes, kidney disease, liver problems, stomach and intestinal disorders, general toxicity and even some highly spiced foods. However, research shows that the main culprits in serious halitosis are **bacteria**.

Your entire intestinal tract, from mouth to anus, is a home for vast numbers of bacteria. In health, they live together in balance and are essential for the wellbeing of the entire body. An imbalance of these germs may occur from poor diet or pollution or medication like antibiotics. The unhealthy bacteria then overgrow, get out of control and result in bad breath. The bad odour is actually caused by volatile sulfur containing substances that these 'bad' bacteria produce.

Apart from the odour they produce, research indicates that an excess of these bacteria in the mouth can promote gum and dental problems, as well as generalised inflammation in the body, and heart and circulatory problems.

Research has also shown that a major area on which these unhealthy bacteria accumulate is at the back of the tongue. These problem germs cannot survive in well-oxygenated areas, so they hide in the thick surface on the back of the tongue and emit the sulfur compounds that cause the offending breath.

THE SOLUTION

Bad breath is a symptom, not a disease, so look for the underlying cause and correct it. Take care of your general health. Your mouth is a mirror of your health. Here are five tips for getting fresher breath.

Brush your tongue

Brushing your teeth is 10 to 20 per cent effective in relieving bad breath; brushing your tongue is about 70 per cent effective. I particularly recommend using a special tongue scraper that allows you to effectively clean the entire tongue especially at the back. These are available in health food stores.

Gargle

The best, cheapest and most effective gargle for bad breath, in my opinion, is hydrogen peroxide. It does not mask the odour but destroys the sulfur-producing bacteria on your tongue by producing lots of oxygen in the bubbles that it creates in your mouth. One to two capfuls of 3 per cent hydrogen peroxide in half a glass of water makes an excellent mouth wash. It is not well promoted as a gargle because drug companies cannot patent it.

Take care of your stomach

Build up of 'bad' bacteria in the stomach causes many problems, from bad breath to peptic ulcers. Replacing the healthy bacteria in the stomach can correct the problem. I recommend a supplement containing acidophilus and bifidus bacteria (Flora Fiber) along with an aloe vera based drink (Herbal Aloe) to promote stomach health.

Cleanse the body

Detoxification of the system, particularly the colon, is also a vital part of the natural approach to correcting bad breath. I use a herbal supplement, colonic irrigation done by a trained colon hydrotherapist and sauna therapy.

Herbs and herbal extracts

Specific herbs naturally sweeten the breath by neutralising the offending sulfur compounds. These include parsley, chlorophyll, sunflower seed oil, spinach extract and cardamom oil. Consult your health food store.

So, cleanse your tongue, mouth, stomach, colon and body and that will cleanse your breath.

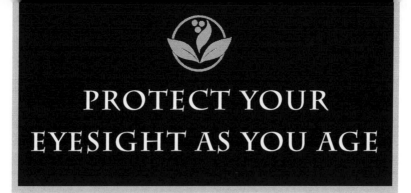

PROTECT YOUR EYESIGHT AS YOU AGE

Fear of losing one's eyesight is one of the common concerns that people have as they age. Of all the five senses, most people would least want to lose their sight. Eyes provide a window to the world. Of course simply aging doesn't mean that your eyesight will diminish, as there are plenty of people in their 80s and beyond who still have good eyesight. However, as you age, changes can indeed occur that may weaken your ability to see.

With your eyesight, as with everything else, 'An ounce of prevention is worth a pound of cure.' Dr Joseph Mercola, a nutritional expert, points out that there are steps you can take to keep your eyes strong and in good health no matter what your age.

TAKE FISH OIL REGULARLY

A fat found in fish called docosahexaenoic acid (DHA) may help protect and promote healthy retinal function. DHA is concentrated in the eye's retina and has been found to be particularly useful in preventing macular degeneration, a leading cause of blindness.

I don't recommend just eating fish, as you need to eat significant quantities of cold water fatty fish like salmon or sardines to get the protection you need. Warm water fish have lower levels of essential fats. Also, we are now concerned about the levels of mercury and other toxins that have been found in fish from oceans, lakes and streams and farm-raised fish. The exception is fish that you have had lab-tested to ensure it is free from contamination.

The best choice, therefore, is to take a high-quality fish oil supplement regularly. Both fish oil and cod liver oil are rich in DHA and EPA, and the fish oils I recommend are purified to the highest standards so you don't need to worry about contaminants.

GET PLENTY OF LUTEIN

Lutein is a carotenoid (one of over 650) found in vegetables and fruits. While beta-carotene, another more famous carotenoid is commonly thought of as important for vision health, lutein may be even more important.

Lutein, which is found in particularly large quantities in green, leafy vegetables, acts as an antioxidant, protecting cells from free radical damage. If you subscribe to a healthy diet, you should receive enough lutein from the food you eat. Unfortunately, most people don't eat enough healthy foods and don't get enough lutein, especially if they rely on fast food as a regular part of their diet.

Adding lutein-rich foods to your diet or taking lutein containing supplements solves the problem. In persons who eat large amounts of fruits and vegetables, it has been found that the risk of age-related macular degeneration decreases some 43 per cent. Excellent sources of lutein include kale, collard greens, spinach, broccoli, Brussels sprouts and egg yolks, particularly raw egg yolks. Egg yolks also have zeaxanthin, another carotenoid, in an equal amount to lutein. Zeaxanthin is likely to be equally as effective as lutein in protecting eyesight.

It is important to note that lutein is an oil-soluble nutrient, and if you merely consume the above vegetables without some oil you can't absorb the lutein. If you are consuming vegetable juice, it would be wise to take your fish oil supplement with the juice to maximise your lutein absorption, as well as the absorption of other important nutrients like vitamin K.

How much lutein is enough? Nutrition experts currently use 6 mg a day as a reliable guideline.

Best food sources of lutein	Per 1/2 cup
Kale, cooked	10 mg
Spinach/callaloo, raw	3.3 mg
Spinach/callaloo, cooked	6.3 mg
Broccoli, raw	1 mg
Broccoli, cooked	1.7 mg
Brussels sprouts, cooked	1.7 mg
Corn, cooked	1.2 mg

EAT DARK COLOURED BERRIES

Not only do berries taste great, but the compounds that give them their dark colour are also great for your health. The European blueberry, also called bilberry, is known to prevent and even reverse macular degeneration, and bioflavonoids from other dark-coloured berries including cranberries and others are also beneficial. They work by strengthening the capillaries that carry nutrients to eye muscles and nerves.

AVOID TRANS-FATS

A diet high in trans-fats appears to contribute to macular degeneration. Trans-fats may interfere with the healthy omega-3 fats in your body, which are extremely important for your eye health.

Trans-fats are commonly found in many processed foods and baked goods, including margarine, shortening, fried foods like French fries, fried chicken and doughnuts, and other foods like cookies, pastries and crackers. Small amounts of trans-fat are almost unavoidable in the modern diet, but we need to keep our intake to a minimum.

DO EYE EXERCISES

There are specific eye exercises that can be done to maintain the strength and function of the small muscles of the eye whose function is important for good eyesight, especially for sharp focus.

 Prevention sure makes a lot more sense than treating the problem after it has occurred.

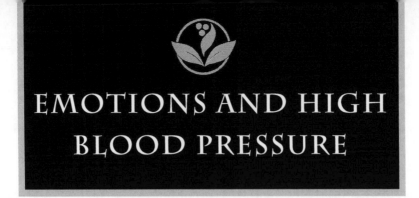

EMOTIONS AND HIGH BLOOD PRESSURE

It is an astonishing fact that, after many decades of medical research, over 95 per cent of the people diagnosed with hypertension are told that they have essential hypertension, meaning that the cause is unknown. In the western world, more visits are made to the doctor for high blood pressure than for any other problem, yet the medical profession still claims ignorance of its underlying cause.

I find this a difficult proposition. I believe that high blood pressure is more of a symptom than a disease. The underlying cause may vary from person to person, but it is important to determine the cause if we are to really deal with the problem. There are often clues to the cause that can facilitate appropriate individual treatment.

WHO GETS HYPERTENSION?

You are 45, slim and fit. You work out at the gym five days each week. You have a wonderful family, a great job and no financial worries. Yet, you have been diagnosed with hypertension and no cause can be found after all the tests have been done. Why?

In his excellent book, *Healing Hypertension*, Dr Samuel Mann of the renowned Hypertension Center of the New York Presbyterian Hospital – Cornell Medical Center, describes four factors that make the development of hypertension likely in an individual:

- Obesity, especially obesity around the waist
- A family history of hypertension

- The severity of stressful life events
- The hiding or suppression of the emotions associated with these stresses.

The first two factors will be well known to the majority of readers, so let us look at the other two: stressful life events and whether we choose to suppress our feelings about them.

STRESSFUL LIFE EVENTS AND HIDDEN EMOTIONS

Here I do not refer to the ordinary stresses of everyday life. Contrary to popular belief, the research shows that, although everyday stress can cause transient increases in blood pressure, it does not usually produce sustained severe elevations in blood pressure. The stresses Dr Mann identifies are the severe stressful life events, often occurring in childhood, which are so overwhelming and potentially destructive that the individual chooses to handle them by hiding away the powerful feelings that surround them. Sometimes the person completely blocks out any memory of the event, while in other cases they can remember the event but express no real feelings about it. A common telltale sign of people in the latter group is when the individual can talk about extremely traumatic issues with no outward sign of emotion. They often claim that they have gotten over it even though they have not addressed it. Those who have blocked their memories often remember very little about their childhood.

My own experience with hard to manage hypertensive patients leads me to agree strongly with Dr Mann. Many people with essential hypertension are manifesting a psychosomatic disorder. As Dr Mann puts it, 'Many people with severe hypertension don't know that their past revisits them every day, whether they feel it or not.' To approach their problem simply with lab tests and powerful drugs is to miss the boat. But the problem must still be addressed. Uncontrolled hypertension from any cause can still kill.

Other disorders associated with hidden emotions

High blood pressure is not the only disorder associated with hidden emotions. A short list of other related conditions which may coexist with hypertension includes:

- Chronic back pain

- Recurrent tension headaches and migraine
- Irregularities of heartbeat
- Irritable Bowel Syndrome
- Sleep disorders, including nightmares and insomnia
- Panic disorder
- Anxiety disorders and hidden depression

GET THE HELP YOU NEED

First, we must remember that not all cases of hypertension are due to suppressed emotions. You may wish to discuss this possibility with an appropriate health care provider. Then, you can consider one or more of the f ollowing therapies:

- Individual or group psychotherapy
- Behavioural techniques – relaxation techniques, stress management, biofeedback and meditation. Along with music therapist Dr Winsome Miller Rowe, I have created a CD entitled *A Time to Relax* which has been a useful tool in the management of stress-induced hypertension.
- Confiding in and connecting with an individual or a group support system
- Hypnotherapy and regression therapy
- Bodywork – emotional release therapy, reflexology, thought field therapy and Reiki.

These modalities may be safely used in conjunction with conventional medication. However, many patients who use these techniques are able to drastically reduce or completely eliminate their need for drug therapy.

Remember, the long-term use of many of the popular drugs for hypertension is not without several potentially serious side effects.

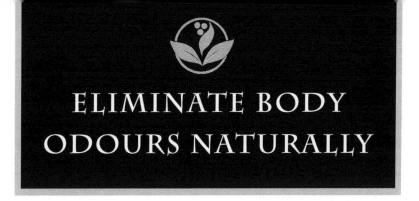

ELIMINATE BODY ODOURS NATURALLY

Body odour is a subject that is quite a sensitive issue for many people. Hundreds of millions of dollars are spent each year on personal care products and deodorants, yet there is almost no discussion about reducing body odour naturally. There is a direct correlation between your health, your diet, your personal habits and the odour produced by your body.

BASICS OF OFFENSIVE BODY ODOURS

What creates the odour?

Conventional wisdom says it is due to bacteria living in your armpits. But think: our entire bodies are covered with bacteria, not just our armpits. And if the bacteria alone were the cause of the odour, you could eliminate body odour by sterilising your armpits with rubbing alcohol or iodine. Try it, if you like, but it won't eliminate the odour. The real cause of armpit odour is the excretion of toxins that your body is trying to get rid of. And by using deodorant products, you block the exit door and force those toxins to stay in your system!

Body odour is something that is strongly affected by what is being emitted by your sweat glands. It may sound simple, but armpits are supposed to perspire. Yet, people go to great lengths to prevent their armpits from sweating by using deodorant products containing toxic chemicals. Many deodorants and antiperspirants are made with aluminium in order to halt the perspiration from your sweat glands. But aluminium is suspected of accumulating in the nervous system and ultimately contributing to nervous system disorders such as Alzheimer's disease.

Your armpits, then, actually have an important health function by getting rid of toxins. That's why you need to keep them open and unclogged by deodorant products. Sweating is good for you.

How the body eliminates toxins

Your body gets rid of toxins through a variety of processes carried out by various organs:

- The intestines excrete undigested food, toxins and bacteria through bowel movements
- The kidneys filter the blood then flush out toxins in the urine
- The lungs remove carbon dioxide and other volatile toxins
- The skin (your body's largest organ) eliminates impurities through sweat

Foods that make you stink

What comes out of your body reflects what you put in the body. Red meat is probably the number one cause of body odour. Modern commercial red meat causes stagnation in the body: it putrefies in the digestive tract and releases lots of toxins into the bloodstream through the large intestine. Some people contend that some vegetarians stink because they wear no deodorant at all. But if a vegetarian has an offensive odour, they are not following a healthy diet even though they are avoiding meat. You can be vegetarian and be extremely unhealthy if you consume a lot of processed foods.

Other foods that cause body odour are manufactured foods containing white flour, added sugars, hydrogenated oils and other processed ingredients.

THE NATURAL WAY TO A HEALTHY ODOUR

The right foods

Shift to a hundred per cent healthy diet made of whole grains, large quantities of green leafy vegetables, fresh fruits, soy products, sprouts, raw nuts and seeds, healthy oils and other similar healthy ingredients. Your body odour will greatly improve because a plant-based diet is an internal deodoriser. The chlorophyll, the fibre and other phytonutrients will cleanse you from the inside out. Some of the best foods for that include aloe, parsley, cilantro, celery and mint. The aromatic herbs – sage, rosemary, thyme and oregano – are also excellent.

Adequate fluids

Drink at least eight glasses of clean water daily to encourage flushing of the kidneys and healthy sweating. Water rich foods – fruit, juices, coconut water, herbal teas, and so on, are also useful.

Internal cleansing

Colon hydrotherapy and herbs like aloe vera, psyllium and milk thistle allow for specific colon cleansing. Periodic fasting on clear fluids only also facilitates internal cleansing. Saunas, sunbaths and vigorous exercise encourage detoxification from the skin. Deep breathing assists cleansing from the lungs.

External cleansing

Regular bathing is essential for a clean body odour. Choose soaps and shampoos that incorporate natural cleaning agents like aloe, natural oils and herbal scents like lavender, rosemary and sage. Skin brushing before bathing with a loofah or skin brush will encourage exfoliation of dead skin cells and open the pores. Good oral hygiene – brushing teeth, flossing and cleaning the tongue – is also an important aspect of external cleansing.

The way to eliminate body odour, then, is not to mask it with unhealthy deodorant products, but to clean your body from both the inside and outside. If you need a deodorant, choose a natural aluminium-free variety.

The things that come out of your body are strong indicators of your level of health. Smell your own armpits and get a sense of what's going on internally. If you can't stand the smell from the outside, just imagine what your body smells like on the inside.

 Remember: Cleanliness is next to Godliness!

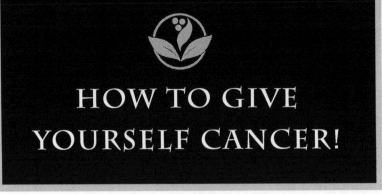

HOW TO GIVE
YOURSELF CANCER!

The second biggest killer of people worldwide is cancer. You may actually be working hard to give yourself cancer and not realise it. It could be breast cancer, prostate cancer, colon cancer or even something like leukemia. By following the instructions below, you can give yourself almost any form of cancer you desire OR you may use the information to protect yourself from this deadly disease.

Keep in mind that everybody potentially has cancer right now. In other words, there are cancerous cells in the body of every person at this very moment. To get diagnosed with cancer, just make sure your immune system is sufficiently suppressed so that your body can't take care of the cancer cells on a regular basis. If you destroy your immune system by an unhealthy lifestyle, then it won't be able to do its job of destroying cancer cells in the body. As a result, cancer can become a full-blown disease in no time. Here are the deadly instructions.

EAT THE WRONG FOODS

The first thing you've got to do is to consume foods containing ingredients that actually promote cancer. One of the most powerful cancer-promoting ingredients is sodium nitrate. This is an ingredient that is added to virtually all packaged meat products including hot dogs, pepperoni, ham, luncheon meat, bacon, sausages and most breakfast meats. It is listed right on the ingredients labels of all of these foods. In order to find sodium nitrate, all you have to do is read the ingredients labels on packaged meat products and purchase them. Then, consume them on a frequent basis and, before long, you will greatly increase your odds of being diagnosed with cancer.

Other ingredients that are suspected of causing cancer include hydro-genated oils, aspartame, saccharin and artificial colouring, to name just a few. A diet that is very high in refined carbohydrates and sugar has also been shown to increase your odds of being diagnosed with cancer, so be sure to get plenty of these foods in your pro-cancer diet. That means eating white bread, sweetened breakfast foods, doughnuts, candy bars, cookies, crackers and sweets of all kinds. Of course, make sure to avoid fruit, vegetables and all forms of fibre.

AVOID ALL SUNLIGHT*

It turns out that natural sunlight provides powerful prevention against cancer. People who get plenty of natural sunlight have a greatly reduced risk of being diagnosed with prostate cancer, breast cancer and many other disorders that aren't cancer-related such as osteoporosis and depression. By staying out of the sun or using sun block and sunscreen every time you're in the sun, you can lower your body's protection against cancer. This is because your body's ability to produce vitamin D is dependent on sun exposure. If you find it difficult to avoid the sun, just get a night-shift job where you work all night and sleep all day. That's a hugely successful pro-cancer strategy.

AVOID ALL PHYSICAL EXERCISE

Exercise helps your body to prevent cancer. Body movement moves lymphatic fluid around, and this is important for your immune system's fight against cancer cells. So do not move: you will increase your odds of being diagnosed with this disease. Deep breathing and rebounding using a trampoline are particularly useful exercises for preventing cancer, so avoid them at all costs!

REMAIN PERMANENTLY STRESSED

All of these strategies for giving yourself cancer have one thing in common: the suppression of your natural immune system. Chronic stress greatly elevates the levels of a stress hormone called cortisol. High cortisol levels powerfully suppress the immune system and may thus promote cancer. So, if you have been doing everything mentioned here, and you want to increase your odds even further, the very best thing you can do is to get yourself physically and mentally stressed out all the time.

SMOKE CIGARETTES

The next thing you can do to give yourself cancer is one of the more obvious things: take up the smoking habit. The more you smoke, the more likely you are to get cancer, especially if you're eating foods with cancer-causing ingredients as discussed above. By smoking, you will multiply the carcinogenic effect of everything else in your life. Before long, you will succeed in your goal of being diagnosed with cancer.

By combining all of these strategies, you should be able to give yourself cancer without much effort and without having to wait too long. Now, all joking aside, why write an article that tells people how to give themselves cancer? The answer is because most people are following this plan right now. Without realising it, they are giving themselves cancer. And when they are diagnosed with cancer, they are distressed and wonder why they are so unfortunate.

At present, statistics indicate that one third of the population will eventually be diagnosed with cancer. This information is presented in this unique way to get the point across that if you don't want to have cancer in your lifetime, you need to get off the cancer plan and start a program that can actually prevent this terrible disease.

---

*An important note about the sun and skin cancer: The great campaign to blame sunlight for causing skin cancer is, I believe, misdirected. Yes, excess exposure of unhealthy skin to sunlight can produce problems. However, when the skin contains high levels of antioxidants, it is not damaged and the whole body benefits in many ways including cancer protection. Rather than using sunblock creams, I recommend using antioxidants like vitamin C both internally and on the skin itself.

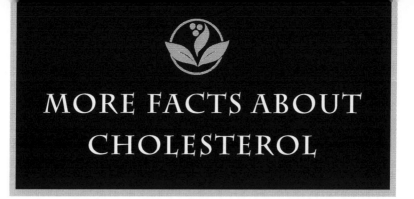

MORE FACTS ABOUT CHOLESTEROL

Everyone, it seems, is now concerned about their cholesterol level. Cholesterol has been made to look like a villain and the drug companies are making immense fortunes from the sale of newer and more expensive cholesterol-lowering drugs. It is important that you know some important facts about cholesterol.

FACT #1

Cholesterol is a natural substance found in every cell and is essential to the structure and function of the body. We could not exist without it. It is not your enemy.

High levels of cholesterol in the blood, especially a type called LDL cholesterol, have been considered a risk factor for cardiovascular disease in general and heart attacks in particular. However, recent research suggests that a high cholesterol level in the blood is only a secondary risk factor. Other blood tests for homocysteine and C-reactive protein are better ways of assessing heart disease risk. Also, low levels of cholesterol are indicators of poor health. As always, maintaining the proper balance is the key.

FACT #2

Most of the cholesterol in the blood, over 70 per cent, is manufactured in the body itself by the liver. Cutting back on high cholesterol foods is a good idea, but this by itself is not an effective way to reduce cholesterol. Cholesterol is so important that the body can easily make it from sugar and other high carbohydrate foods. Thus, someone on a totally cholesterol-free diet can still have an elevation of cholesterol in the blood. You do not have to eat fatty foods to have high cholesterol.

Many of the 'low cholesterol foods' being advertised are so full of sugar and carbohydrates that, as far as lowering your blood cholesterol is concerned, you are 'swapping black dog for monkey' when you eat them.

FACT #3

The popular cholesterol-lowering drugs act primarily by interfering with the function of the liver (I call them slow liver poisons), and their use is associated with a long list of potential side effects. People on these medications are required to do regular liver tests to detect signs of liver damage. Drinking alcohol also lowers cholesterol by damaging the liver, but I hope that no one would consider using it for that purpose. Drugs to lower cholesterol should in my opinion be considered as a last resort, and not prescribed as readily as they are now.

If I wanted to use a 'drug', I would recommend a 'natural' one made from the sugar cane plant and developed in Cuba called Arteriomixol. It does as good or better a job than the conventional ones and does not poison the liver. It may even improve your sex life.

FACT #4

Lifestyle changes play a major role in normalising cholesterol levels. Lifestyle modification, therefore, should be the first and most important part of any program for lowering cholesterol. This includes the following:

Diet

Diet is very important, but do not just focus on low cholesterol foods as is the fashion. A diet high in fibre, low in animal fats and low in simple carbohydrates (especially sugar and flour) is ideal.

Weight control

Correcting obesity, particularly losing fat from around the waist, is vital to lowering cholesterol.

Exercise

Exercise, as little as 30 minutes of brisk walking, four times per week, assists in lowering cholesterol. It also benefits overall health in many other ways.

Stress management

Stress itself can elevate cholesterol levels as the body manufactures more cholesterol when stressed. Stress management techniques like relaxation exercises, meditation, yoga and tai chi are an important part of a holistic health care approach.

FACT#5

There are several nutritional supplements and herbs that are effective agents for dealing with the cholesterol problem. In addition, they are not only safe but have many other health benefits as well.

- **The antioxidants** – The vitamins A,C, E and selenium (I call them the ACES) comprise the antioxidants. Cholesterol is really dangerous and unhealthy only when it is oxidised by molecules called free radicals. Antioxidants protect cholesterol from oxidisation. Vitamin E is particularly important in this regard. Herbal antioxidants like garlic, schizandra, rosemary, pycnogenol and ginger are also extremely useful.

- **Fish oils** – These are high in omega-3 fatty acids which lower cholesterol.

- **Soy and oats** – These are foods high in soluble fibre which also lower cholesterol. I recommend a soy-based shake every day.

- **Niacin (vitamin B$_3$)** – In adequate dosages, niacin effectively lowers cholesterol. Use a form of niacin called niacinate to prevent flushing of the skin and have a holistic doctor supervise the dosage.

So start today to manage your cholesterol the natural way.

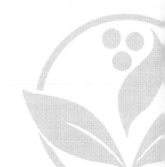

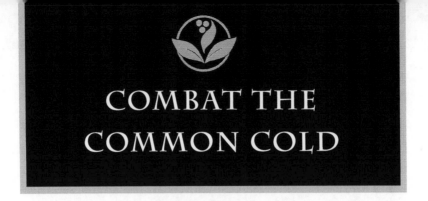

COMBAT THE COMMON COLD

When there are heavy rains and damp conditions, one can expect to see more people coming down with a cold. The 'common cold' is caused by a wide variety of viruses that infects the upper respiratory tract, the nasal passages, the sinuses and the throat. We are all constantly exposed to these viruses and the fact that we do not have colds all the time is because our immune system is protecting us. Frequent colds suggest a weak immune system.

Maintaining a healthy immune system is the primary way to protect yourself against frequent colds. But what do you do if you get a cold? With a healthy, functioning immune system, a cold should not last longer than three to four days. Most conventional cold medications are designed to suppress the symptoms of a cold, but there are natural ways to assist the body to recover. Here are five tips to help your body to resist a cold naturally.

REST

The value of sleep and rest during a common cold cannot be over emphasised. At the first sign of a cold, decrease your activities and rest as much as possible. Avoid stress. During deep sleep the body releases powerful immunity-enhancing substances that increase your healing capacity. Relaxation and deep breathing exercises are very useful.

INCREASE FLUID INTAKE

Drink lots of liquids. When the membranes of the respiratory tract are dehydrated, cold viruses have an ideal environment to grow in. Moist, well-hydrated membranes decrease your risk of acquiring these viral infections.

The choice of liquid is vital. Research has shown that very sweet drinks reduce the ability of the white blood cells to kill germs because of the high sugar content. So, even fruit juices should be greatly diluted. Water, vegetable juices, herbal teas and vegetable broth are ideal.

TAKE VITAMIN C AND HERBAL ANTIOXIDANTS

Vitamin C at a dosage of six grams daily has been shown to reduce the severity and duration of a cold by 20 per cent. It should be taken in divided dosages (that is, two or three times daily instead of all at once), and the quantity gradually increased to the point where you begin to have loose stools. This is an indication that you have passed your optimal dosage. Simply reduce the dosage to a level where bowel activity returns to normal.

The Chinese herb schizandra and the local herb rosemary are particularly useful in boosting the immune system to fight off the cold virus. They are available as tablets and should be taken in high dosages (that is, two or three times the dose recommended on the label) at the first sign of a cold.

USE ECHINACEA

This herb is famous as a herbal antibiotic and antiviral agent. Taking 900 milligrams of Echinacea root daily significantly reduces the symptoms of the common cold. In 1994, German doctors handed out 2.5 million prescriptions for Echinacea for the common cold. It is available as tablets, tinctures and teas.

SUCK ON ZINC LOZENGES

Many studies have demonstrated that zinc lozenges greatly reduce the severity and duration of cold symptoms. They should be sucked like sweets every two to four hours. The best zinc lozenges for the cold contain the amino acid glycine.

WASH YOUR HANDS

Avoid putting your hands near your eyes, nose or mouth unless you have washed them. Most bacteria and germs are spread from a surface to your hands and from your hands to your face. Few germs are transmitted through the air. Clean shared objects that are used by several people during the day more often, for example, phones, keyboards, steering wheels, office equipment and other items.

There you have it, five simple, safe, natural interventions that can reduce the misery of the common cold. Try to prevent the cold by keeping your immune system strong.

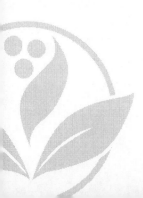

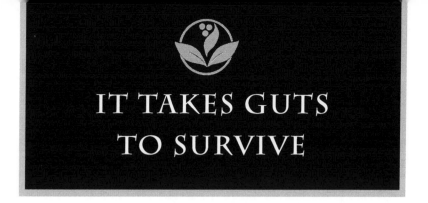

IT TAKES GUTS
TO SURVIVE

'Take care of your gut and the body will look after the rest', is a saying that I first heard from an older English doctor a long time ago. Many years later I have come to appreciate the great wisdom in that saying. The term 'gut' refers to the intestinal tract, a passage well over 20 feet long, which starts at the mouth and ends at the anus.

YOUR GUT CONTROLS YOUR NUTRITION

No matter how nutritious your diet is, the food must first be digested and absorbed so that the nutrients can be transported to all the tissues of the body to provide your cells with cellular nutrition. Without a properly functioning intestinal tract (gut), a lot of the nutrients in your food may end up in the toilet bowl. That is why many people who take vitamins often complain that they have not noticed any difference in their health and wellbeing. That is why I recommend a nutritional program called the Cellular Nutrition Program, which ensures that you not only take in the right nutrients, but that they are readily absorbed and easily available for your cells to utilise.

YOUR GUT PROTECTS YOU

Most people put between three to five pounds of solids and liquids (often mislabeled 'food') into their bodies every day. Some of this stuff is strange and foreign to the body and can be downright harmful. This includes food additives, chemical contaminants like insecticides, hormones, antibiotics and other drugs, and germs of various types. The gut has very sophisticated defense systems to protect us from harm. There are more immune system cells surrounding the gut than any other system in the human body. Despite this, we so often overburden our guts that food allergies and intestinal infections are extremely common, often debilitating and sometimes life threatening. The young are particularly vulnerable because their immune systems are not yet fully developed; millions of children still die each year from intestinal infections.

YOUR GUT IS ALIVE

Your gut is not just an empty tube that food passes through. It is a complex ecosystem populated by billions and billions of bacteria. There are more bacteria in your gut than there are cells in your body. There are many different types of bacteria in your intestines, some 'good' guys and some 'bad' guys. They live together in a delicate balance and are extremely important, not only to the gut, but also to the health of the entire body. Many things can produce an imbalance of these germs, for example, drugs like antibiotics, too much sugar or too little fibre in the diet, or some dairy products. This creates a condition called dysbiosis with symptoms like gas, bloating, gastritis, stomach ulcers, cramps and diarrhoea and/or constipation.

Many seemingly unrelated illnesses like arthritis, allergies, nervous system disorders and autoimmune diseases may be related to disturbances in the functioning of your gut. Here are a few tips for a healthy gut:

- Have good balanced nutrition with an emphasis on natural high fibre foods. Be particularly wary of chemical food additives, excess sugar and dairy products. I particularly recommend the soy-based Cellular Nutrition Program.

- Employ some form of regular cleansing, particularly colon cleansing. I use a natural herbal combination sometimes combined with colon hydrotherapy.

- Take aloe vera. It is extremely good for the entire digestive system. I use a convenient, pleasant tasting drink made from aloe and other herbs. It is healing, gently cleansing and soothing. I have not prescribed any 'gas medicine' for my patients for almost a decade, but use aloe exclusively.

- Put back the good bacteria in the gut along with additional fibre. I use a supplement called Flora Fiber, which contains acidophilus and lacto-bacillus bacteria in a fibre blend. Natural yogurt is also useful.

- Eat smaller frequent meals. Try not to overburden your intestines at any one time. As my grandfather used to say, you should leave the dining table feeling that you could have had a little bit more.

- Learn good stress management. Many gut problems are stress related.

 Remember, take care of your gut and it will take care of you.

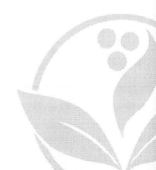

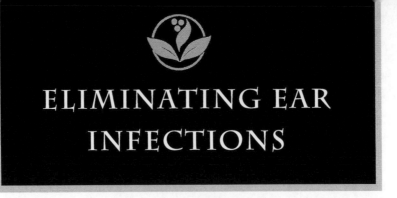

ELIMINATING EAR INFECTIONS

Ear infections are extremely common. Many children (and their distressed parents) suffer from recurrent bouts of middle ear infections called otitis media. These infections cause tremendous pain, misery and expense, and may be accompanied by serious complications. The first line of conventional treatment, antibiotics, used repeatedly, can itself produce side effects by weakening the child's immune system and by creating antibiotic resistant germs. If antibiotics do not seem to be controlling the problem, then even more invasive and expensive methods are usually recommended: draining the middle ear by inserting plastic tubes through the ear drum or having the tonsils and adenoids removed if they have become enlarged.

Let's look at some ways to prevent ear infections in your child and you:

BREASTFEED

Breast-fed infants get fewer ear infections than bottle-fed ones. Breast milk provides immune factors from the mother called antibodies that assist the child in fighting infections.

AVOID DAIRY PRODUCTS

The proteins in cow's milk disturb the immune system in many children. Dairy can also stimulate the production of excess mucus and congestion that set the stage for infection. If your child gets recurring ear infections or colds, replace dairy products with soy milk and soy products.

STRENGTHEN THE IMMUNE SYSTEM

A cold can often bring on an ear infection. Strengthen the immune system by ensuring your child eats a healthy diet, drinks lots of water, gets enough rest and washes his or her hands frequently. A good multivitamin/herbal supplement containing antioxidants like vitamin C, schizandra, rosemary, garlic and pycnogenol are extremely useful and safe for building the immune system. If a cold threatens, additional vitamin C and echinacea are recommended.

DO NOT SMOKE

Children whose parents smoke get a lot more ear infections than those whose parents do not smoke. Also, do not let other people smoke around your children. To make it even worse, if you smoke, it increases the chance that your child will take up smoking later.

AVOID GETTING WATER IN THE EAR

Adults will more often get an infection of the ear canal (otitis externa) due to a bacteria or fungus. It causes pain and itching and is usually related to water in the ear from swimming or even washing your hair. A good natural prevention if you get water in your ear is to mix equal parts of rubbing alcohol and white vinegar and put a few drops in each ear. This will help to kill any germs and to remove the moisture from the ear. In severe cases, your doctor may need to prescribe a short course of antimicrobial eardrops.

I have seen these measures relieve and prevent a lot of suffering and expense for many families. Please make use of these simple 'ounces of prevention'.

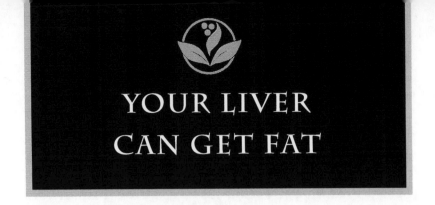

YOUR LIVER CAN GET FAT

As the obesity epidemic accelerates, medical experts are discovering more and more health problems associated with just being too fat. Your liver can also get too fat.

The liver is one of the body's most important organs. It manufactures many important substances, plays a major role in our digestive processes while detoxifying and clearing toxins from the blood. Normally, the liver can handle a lot of abuse and has a tremendous ability to regenerate itself after damage and stress.

FATTY LIVER

Unfortunately, most people, including many doctors, are unaware of a liver problem that researchers say is now the commonest liver disorder in developed countries. It is estimated to affect almost a quarter of the American population. It is called Nonalcoholic Fatty Liver Disease (NAFLD). The name speaks for itself: it is an accumulation of fat in the liver, occupying over 10 per cent of the organ, in people who drink little or no alcohol. The latter distinction is important as, in the past, a fatty liver was typically associated with alcohol abuse.

Who is at risk?

The disease can strike anyone, but certain persons are at high risk. They include:

- **The obese.** Ninety per cent of obese individuals are at risk of damaging their liver. Even more important is where the excess fat is stored. Fat around the waist (truncal obesity) is not just stored under the skin. It surrounds and infiltrates the abdominal organs. This is particularly true for the liver where fat globules actually enter the liver cells and damage them.

- **The diabetic.** Fifty per cent of diabetics have NAFLD, and just about all obese diabetics will have the disorder. Insulin resistance, a condition associated with Type 2 diabetes and obesity, seems to play a major role in this liver disease.

- **Persons with high cholesterol levels.** A very high percentage of individuals with elevated LDL cholesterol and triglycerides have excess fat infiltrating their livers.

- **The elderly.** The prevalence of NAFLD rises with age and recent studies show that over 65 per cent of persons over age 80 have this condition. Unfortunately, obese children may also already have fatty livers.

All these people are prone to a condition called insulin resistance in which there is an elevation of the levels of insulin in the blood. This elevation of insulin (hyperinsulinemia) leads to a fatty liver.

What are the symptoms?

Like diabetes and high blood pressure, this liver condition is often initially silent, but causes life-threatening problems many years later. In some cases, patients may have only non-specific complaints like low energy, fatigue, malaise and mild upper abdominal pain. Laboratory tests for liver function may or may not reveal any abnormality. Later in the progression of the disease, signs of inflammation of the liver (hepatitis), cirrhosis, liver failure or liver cancer may develop.

Can NAFLD be treated or prevented?

Conventional medicine does not have a specific drug or treatment for this problem. However, the condition can be largely prevented and sometimes reversed by nutritional and lifestyle modification through:

- **Weight loss.** Losing weight with a nutritionally sound weight-loss program will result in a significant reduction of excess fat in the liver. I have found a low carbohydrate Cellular Nutrition program effective in this regard. Correcting truncal obesity is an essential part of any treatment plan.

- **Controlling blood sugar levels.** Maintaining normal blood sugar levels is also critical in managing this problem.

- **Antioxidant supplementation.** Take vitamins A, C and E, selenium, alpha lipoic acid, Coenzyme Q10 and glutathione (Immunucal).

- **Detoxification programs.** These will help to relieve the toxic burden on an already compromised liver. The herb milk thistle is particularly useful in this regard. Alcohol and other liver toxins must be absolutely avoided.

- **Soy products.** Soybeans contain a form of phosphatidylcholine, which has been shown in some studies to halt the progress of liver damage in NAFLD.

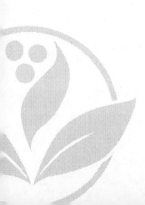

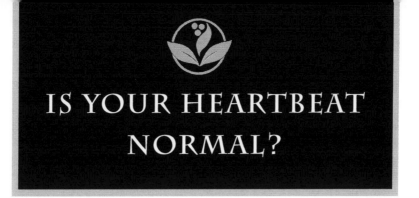

IS YOUR HEARTBEAT NORMAL?

Heart disease is the world's number one killer. Let us look at one important aspect of heart function – the heartbeat. The human heart pumps over 100,000 times every day, or about 70 times a minute, every hour of the day, every day of the year. No man-made pump could function with this level of efficiency. We are indeed fearfully and wonderfully made. However, your heart's rhythm is not always as regular as clockwork.

In truth, we all have some measure of irregularity to our heartbeats, and no one's heart rhythm is perfectly regular. Mild beat-to-beat variation may, in fact, indicate good overall health. Physically fit athletes, for example, have the greatest degree of heartbeat variation. However, your heart's rate/rhythm can exceed healthy limits of variation. This condition is called an **arrhythmia**.

Some arrhythmias are benign and are simply an annoyance (albeit a frightening one when your heart feels as though it is jumping and racing). Others, however, can be life threatening. How can you tell the difference? What can you do to promote a healthy heartbeat?

UNDERSTANDING THE HEARTBEAT

Several basic facts can help us understand whether dangers are present or we are just experiencing a harmless irregularity of the heart.

Heart rate

Normal heart rate ranges widely, depending on age, fitness level, mood, physical activity, and fluid and drug intake. The range considered normal and safe is 50 to 99 beats per minute. Rates at the lower end suggest fitness, as in the case of long-distance runners, although heart rate can also decline with age.

Sustained rates at the high end (above 85 beats per minute) can be due to problems in the heart itself or may suggest other processes such as dehydration, thyroid disorders, infections and anxiety.

Heart rhythm

The rhythm of the heart is also important. An irregular heartbeat may present as a feeling of the heart skipping a beat or a sudden racing of the heart. A special test called an electrocardiogram (ECG or EKG), can be performed by your doctor to carefully examine your heart's rhythm.

Despite changes in rate and rhythm, the heart must maintain its essential function: to pump blood throughout the body. If the heart beats too slowly, too quickly, or too irregularly, it may struggle to do its job. When the heart's blood output diminishes, we can become lightheaded, breathless, and even lose consciousness. In the worst case, some arrhythmias can be fatal. Heart rates that are less than or greater than the normal range of 50 to 99 beats per minute are clearly abnormal and should be addressed by a physician.

MAINTAINING A HEALTHY HEARTBEAT NATURALLY

Having checked with your doctor to exclude heart disease or other medical disorders, there are natural supplements that you can take to help promote a healthy heartbeat. These are listed below.

Fish oil

Inexpensive, safe and effective, fish oil is the closest thing we have to an ideal anti-arrhythmia drug. Fish oil is the most concentrated source of omega-3 fatty acids, known technically as EPA and DHA. Fish oil not only sharply reduces the frequency of irregular beats, it also diminishes the likelihood of death from dangerous arrhythmias. Fish oil achieves all this without significant side effects, an advantage which is lacking in every prescribed anti-arrhythmia medication.

A secondary source of omega-3 fatty acids, called ALA, is found in flaxseed, walnuts and canola oil. When humans ingest ALA, however, only 10 per cent of it is converted into active EPA or DHA that helps the heart.

Magnesium

Magnesium is a crucial nutrient that helps to ensure the proper functioning of the human body. Unfortunately, on average, we consume far less than the daily recommended dietary allowance. Low magnesium levels promote abnormal heart rhythms.

Moreover, research has demonstrated that our magnesium intake is dropping precipitously as we consume even greater amounts of magnesium-depleted processed foods (for example, alcohol, white sugar, high fructose corn syrup, white flour and highly salted foods) and drinks.

Soft drinks (both diet and regular), for example, are manufactured using water that is essentially devoid of magnesium. These sodas also contain phosphates that prevent magnesium from being absorbed in the intestinal tract. To make matters worse, more of us are drinking bottled water many brands of which contain little or no magnesium. Coffee is also a magnesium depleted beverage.

Because low magnesium tissue levels are so common, everyone with an irregular heartbeat should practise magnesium supplementation. They should also eat lots of magnesium-rich foods, such as nuts, beans and green leafy vegetables.

Coenzyme Q10

Coenzyme Q10 (CoQ10) is a substance found in the mitochondria (energy generators) of the body's cells, especially the heart cells. Arrhythmias commonly occur when there is an abnormal weakness of the heart muscle. Research has shown that CoQ10 supplementation can benefit people with weakened heart muscles and may help lessen the risk of arrhythmias. It is a safe, natural and effective nutritional agent that is virtually free of side effects.

Hawthorn

Hawthorn (Crataegus oxyacantha) is a small, native European tree whose berries, flowers and leaves have been used therapeutically since the Middle Ages as an aid in treating heart failure. Recent studies suggest that it helps to correct an irregular heartbeat.

Avoid excess stimulants

Excess amounts of caffeine (found in coffee, some teas and soft drinks), nicotine, alcohol, cocaine, marijuana, as well as a long list of prescription and non-prescription drugs can all cause an irregular heartbeat. Be moderate in your use of stimulants.

Manage stress

Finally, poorly managed stress is a common cause of irregular heartbeat. The classic panic attack is an exaggerated stress reaction in which the sufferer commonly experiences a racing heart, difficulty in breathing and sometimes chest pain. Practice relaxation techniques and learn to manage stress in a healthy way.

 Take care of your heart and it will take care of you.

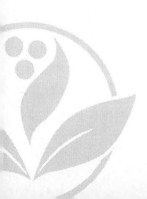

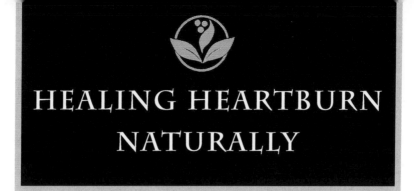

HEALING HEARTBURN NATURALLY

WHAT IS HEARTBURN?

Interestingly, heartburn has nothing to do with the heart. It is a painful burning sensation in the throat and chest. The pain often rises in the chest and may then radiate to the neck or throat. It results from the reflux of juices (containing hydrochloric acid) from the stomach into the oesophagus or (gullet). The new medical term for it is **GERD** (**G**astro-**E**sophageal **R**eflux **D**isease).

About 10 per cent of the population has heartburn daily, and in most cases, it's mild and temporary. Some have chronic heartburn that hits them day and night. Those who are coping with heartburn need to be aware that they may be in danger of developing esophageal cancer if their symptoms become chronic. As with peptic ulcers, conventional medicine has focused on acid as the villain and the cause of the problem. As such, a vast array of powerful, expensive and dangerous drugs are prescribed along with the old-fashioned antacids for this disorder.

ACID IS NOT THE PROBLEM

Contrary to what virtually every television advertisement about heartburn tells you, neutralising stomach acid is not the answer. The stomach is meant to produce acid. This acid is essential in preparing the food for digestion and it also destroys unhealthy germs present in the food we eat. Taking drugs and antacids that block or neutralise the acid is in fact working against the body's natural function. The real problem is that the acid is getting into the wrong place – the oesophagus.

Between the stomach and the oesophagus, there is a sphincter (valve) that prevents the acidic stomach juices from refluxing or flowing backwards into the oesophagus. Proper digestion involves a process which creates a high concentration of acid in the stomach while tightening the sphincter and protecting the oesophagus. Several things can cause this valve to malfunction and result in heartburn. Therefore, it is important to treat the underlying cause so that the problem can disappear. Apart from the fact that antacid drugs simply treat the symptoms of heartburn rather than the underlying causes, they can also contribute to the problem. If you try to kill off stomach acids with antacid drugs, the body stops protecting the oesophagus from the acids that cause heartburn. The sphincter relaxes and allows some stomach acid to slip past, which irritates the oesophagus, and causes heartburn. For many people, this sets off a vicious cycle in which they take more antacids which, in turn, results in more heartburn.

THE FIVE Cs OF HEARTBURN

Here are some natural approaches that I have found both safe and effective in dealing with heartburn. I call them the five Cs of heartburn.

Change your diet

Avoid fatty foods, alcohol, coffee, highly-spiced foods and any other foods that bring on heartburn. Do not eat large meals, especially at night. Remain upright and active after eating and allow the food to digest and the stomach to empty before lying down.

Correct obesity

Obesity, especially around the waist, promotes acid reflux. A weight loss program using frequent, small, low carbohydrate meals is excellent for this condition. The weight-loss program I know is called ShapeWorks. It is particularly useful for people with heartburn.

Check your drug use

Many drugs frequently prescribed for common problems such as arthritis, hypertension, diabetes, pain, anxiety and even stomach problems can themselves cause heartburn. Discuss with your doctor the possibility of reducing or eliminating your need for medication.

Control stress

The activity of the stomach is controlled by one of the largest nerves in the body (the vagus nerve) that comes directly from the brain. Chronic stress, anxiety, nervous tension and depression can all contribute to heartburn, and drugs often prescribed for these problems can make it worse. Irritable Bowel Syndrome (IBS) is a classic example of how the nervous system can affect the digestive system. Learn to manage these problems in as holistic a way as possible. Simple relaxation and stress management exercises can be very useful.

Choose natural alternatives

I have not prescribed a drug for heartburn in over 12 years. Instead, I recommend the following for my patients:

- **Aloe vera** – An aloe vera juice and chamomile combination is very effective in dealing with acid reflux. The aloe extract restores and heals the normal protective lining of the stomach and oesophagus, while the chamomile relaxes the stomach and reduces acid reflux.

- **Probiotics** – Healthy bacteria like Lactobacillus acidophilus, combined with fibre, assist in rapidly healing and restoring normal function to the oesophagus and stomach as well as the entire intestinal tract. This combination is available in tablet form as a nutritional supplement (Flora Fiber). When taken with the aloe vera juice extract, it does wonders for heartburn.

 Remember, it is always better to deal with the underlying problem rather than just treat the symptoms.

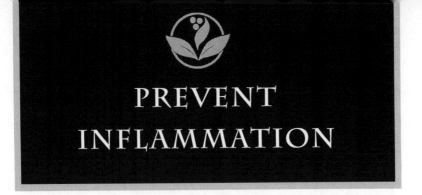

PREVENT INFLAMMATION

A large number of diseases are due to inflammation. In fact the suffix 'itis' at the end of so many medical words indicates inflammation. Arthritis, for example, means an inflammation of the joints, appendicitis indicates an inflammation of the appendix and gastritis means an inflammation of the stomach. Inflammation produces pain, swelling, heat and loss of function. Chronic inflammation inflicts devastating effects on health. A long list of common but seemingly unrelated health problems, including asthma and allergies, heart disease, kidney failure, stroke and Alzheimer's disease, all have their genesis in inflammation. In addition, many of the 'diseases of old age' are simply the result of long-standing inflammation.

A vast number of drugs are taken to simply suppress or control these symptoms. They are called anti-inflammatory drugs. These drugs may initially be effective in easing the pain or reducing the swelling, but they do not deal with the underlying problem, they simply control the symptom. What is worse, they have major side effects especially when taken for prolonged periods: your stomach might develop bleeding ulcers or your kidneys may become damaged.

FOUR STEP PROGRAM

The good news is that your body is designed with the ability to control, reverse and even prevent inflammation. This four step program can help.

Step 1: Proper nutrition

As I have said a million times, you are what you eat. Certain foods promote inflammation while others prevent and relieve it. The following foods should be avoided:

- Fatty red meat, fried foods, organ meats like liver and kidney, dairy products and egg yolks (these contain pro-inflammatory substances)

- Rice, pasta, refined flour products like dumplings, crackers and white bread (these elevate blood sugar levels and create hormonal imbalance)

- Sugar, excess sweet fruits and fruit juices (these elevate blood sugar)

- Food flavourings, preservatives and artificial food colourings.

The following foods should be emphasized:

- Mackerel, salmon and other cold water fish

- Fresh vegetables and certain fruit (such as fruit that is not very sweet like grapefruit, berries, melons and papaya)

- Virgin olive oil and olives, flaxseed, flaxseed oil and avocados

- Oatmeal, nuts, seeds and whole grain.

Step 2: Cleanse and detoxify the body

It is important to look for and clear up any sites of chronic infection in the body. Particular attention should be paid to the mouth (teeth and gums), the sinuses, the nails (fungal infections) and the skin. You may need the assistance of your medical practitioner for this. Natural detoxification programs using herbs, colonic irrigation, steam or saunas, massage and liquid fasts are very effective. These may be necessary at regular intervals.

Step 3: Supplements

A program of vitamin and mineral supplements is advised. I recommend following a Cellular Nutrition plan. In addition, there are some specific anti-inflammatory supplements that will assist the body in correcting the imbalance that produced the inflammation. These include:

- fish oil capsules (use a high quality variety from several different fish)

- the antioxidants (vitamins A, C, E and selenium)

- herbs: nettle leaf extract, boswellia and curcumin

- DHEA and vitamin E.

Step 4: Stress management

Poorly managed, chronic stress produces certain chemical imbalances in the body that promote inflammatory responses. Learning to identify the stressors in one's life and developing effective stress management techniques are extremely important aspects of any program for controlling inflammation. Develop an emotional and spiritual support system. Healthy relationships, prayer, meditation and other spiritual practices can greatly facilitate the healing process.

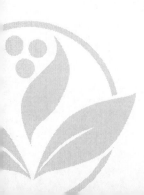

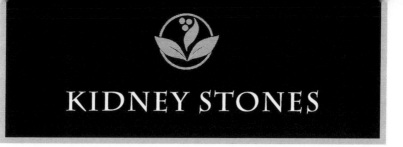

KIDNEY STONES

Your kidneys are bean-shaped organs, each about the size of your fist. They are located near the middle of your back, just below the rib cage, one on each side of the spine.

Your kidneys are sophisticated trash collectors. Every day, they filter about 200 quarts of blood to create about 2 quarts of waste products and extra water. This becomes urine, which flows from your kidneys to your bladder through tubes called ureters. Your bladder stores the urine until it is convenient for you to void it.

WHAT ARE KIDNEY STONES?

A kidney stone is a solid piece of material that forms in a kidney out of substances in the urine. Most kidney stones are made from calcium oxalate, that is, calcium combined with oxalic acid. Several other types of stones occur but they are more rare.

A stone may stay in the kidney or break loose and travel down the urinary tract. A small stone may pass all the way out of the body without causing too much pain. A larger stone may get stuck in the passage, block the flow of urine and cause great pain.

Kidney stones may lie dormant in your kidneys for a long time and may only be discovered when they show up on an X-ray. They can, however, cause problems such as backache, urinary tract infections, blood in the urine, kidney damage and the dreaded *renal colic*.

Renal colic is the excruciating pain experienced when a kidney stone is being passed along the ureter. Experts claim that this is the most severe pain known to man (and woman). It usually originates in the loin areas but may radiate down into the genitals. One sufferer said that it felt as if someone had plunged a knife into his lower back and was continuously twisting and turning it in his flesh. Not an experience you would wish to have! So what can be done to prevent it?

PREVENTING KIDNEY STONES

Here are some suggestions for preventing kidney stones.

- **Avoid dehydration.** There is ample evidence to suggest that a major cause of kidney stones is dehydration. The more concentrated your urine, the greater the risk of stone formation. Therefore, drink more water to create larger quantities of a more dilute urine.

  Try to drink half an ounce of water for each pound of your body weight. Drinking lots of water helps to flush away the substances that form stones in the kidneys. Distilled water with lime or lemon juice is particularly helpful. Other useful fluids include coconut water, cranberry juice, watermelon juice and dandelion tea.

- **Consume less meat.** Professor W.G. Robertson from the Medical Research Council in Leeds, England, is one of the foremost experts in diet and kidney stones. His research shows that consuming animal protein will greatly increase your risk of forming kidney stones.

  Why is this so? When enough foods containing animal protein are consumed, the concentration of calcium and oxalate in the urine increases sharply within a few hours. When the kidneys are under a persistent long-term assault from increased calcium and oxalate, kidney stones are most likely to result.

  Robertson published studies that showed how patients with recurrent kidney stones could resolve their problem by simply shifting their diet away from animal proteins. The worldwide problem of kidney stone formation appears to be particularly aggravated by a high consumption of dairy products.

- **Take supplements.** Supplementation with vitamin B_6 and magnesium lowers the levels of calcium and oxalate in the urine and thus helps to reduce kidney stone formation.

FLUSHING OUT KIDNEY STONES

Conventional treatments for kidney stones involve expensive, invasive surgical interventions or high-tech techniques to shatter large stones with sound waves.

Some inexpensive, low-tech, non-invasive approaches are worth considering. They seek to assist the body to flush out smaller kidney stones in a non-toxic way.

Kidney flush #1

Required ingredients

- Six 12-ounce cans of Coca Cola or a 2-litre bottle of Coca Cola.

  The high phosphoric acid content of this beverage is a powerful catalyst for dissolving your kidney stones. It will dissolve corrosion on your battery terminals too. I do not recommend this drink for general use.

- 6–8 ounces of fresh asparagus (canned or frozen works too)

- Distilled water

Procedure

1. Over the course of 2 hours, drink the 72 ounces of Coca Cola

2. Steam or quickly boil the asparagus. Process in the blender until well puréed

3. Within 5 minutes of drinking the last 12 ounces, eat the asparagus purée. Instead of just gulping it down, try to mix the purée well with your saliva

   Try to keep from urinating for as long as possible. The remedy begins working immediately and, within a few hours, you should begin to pass the stones through your urine as sand-like particles.

Kidney flush #2 (Celery seed remedy)

(WARNING: This remedy should not be used by pregnant women.)

Required ingredients

- 2 tablespoons of celery seeds

- 2 cups of water

Procedure

1. Bring the water to a boil.

2. Add the celery seeds and cook until soft.

3. Remove mixture from heat and strain off seeds from the water.

4. Drink the tea – half a cup every hour over the course of 2 hours.

As with the first remedy, try to keep from urinating for as long as possible.

 So, again I suggest: An ounce of prevention is worth a ton of painful and expensive cure.

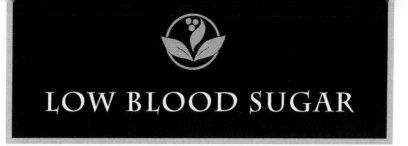

LOW BLOOD SUGAR

The technical term for a low blood sugar level is hypoglycaemia. The 'sugar' referred to is a substance called glucose. Glucose is the main fuel that our cells burn to create the energy for our body to function properly. A healthy body keeps the level of glucose in the blood within very narrow limits, as too high or too low a level of blood sugar can severely disturb many important functions of the body.

Much attention is paid to high levels of blood sugar, the outstanding feature of the common disease diabetes. But low blood sugar can be even more common and more dangerous. Both high and low blood sugar are, in fact, aspects of the same problem, described by doctors as dysglycaemia. I believe that both these conditions have common causes and similar solutions.

Excess carbohydrates in the body, particularly refined sugars, will cause the body to secrete excess amounts of the hormone called insulin. This can result in a fall in blood sugar, sometimes to dangerously low levels. Many people live with their blood sugar swinging dangerously from high to low. This situation actually sets the stage for the development of diabetes later in life. Early detection and correction of this situation can prevent the onset of diabetes. It is important to recognise that diabetes starts to develop many years before it is officially diagnosed and low blood sugar is often an early sign of impending diabetes.

COMMON CAUSES OF LOW BLOOD SUGAR

- Poor eating habits with missed, late or inadequate meals
- Eating carbohydrate-rich foods, such as starches and simple sugars
- Taking diabetic medication, both insulin and tablets
- Alcohol consumption, which can contribute to liver and pancreas diseases

COMMON SYMPTOMS AND SIGNS

- Sweating and trembling
- Palpitations (that is, a pounding heart)
- Hunger, nausea or vomiting
- Anxiety and panic
- Speech difficulty and poor coordination
- Inability to concentrate
- Headaches
- Confusion, drowsiness, coma and even death

Hypoglycaemia Questionnaire

Questions	Yes	No
Do you crave sweets?		
Do you feel irritable and tired if you miss a meal?		
Do you feel tired an hour or so after a meal?		
Do you get dizzy when you stand too quickly?		
Is your memory or concentration poor?		
Do you experience blurred vision?		
Are you frequently anxious, nervous or shaky?		
Do you have bouts of depression or mood swings?		
Do you get fatigued during the afternoon?		
Are you overweight?		
Total		

Score
4 or less positive answers: **hypoglycaemia unlikely.**
4 to 8 positive answers: **hypoglycaemia is possible.**
8 or more positive answers: **hypoglycaemia very likely.**

SOME EFFECTS OF HYPOGLYCAEMIA

Although conventional medicine took a relatively long time to accept hypoglycaemia as an important health issue, research has shown that it has far reaching health consequences. Some of these are listed below.

Syndrome X/Metabolic syndrome

These are terms used to describe a combination of common conditions including diabetes, high blood pressure, heart and circulatory disorders, elevated cholesterol and triglyceride levels and obesity. Although modern medicine treats these conditions with a variety of different medicines as if they are all unrelated, they all have a common basis – too much insulin in the blood. Hypoglycaemia is a common warning sign of the development of these conditions.

Brain dysfunction

When the brain is starved of glucose, it malfunctions. Dizziness, headache, clouded vision, blunted mental activity, emotional instability and confusion can result. There is even a strong, but controversial link between hypoglycaemia and criminal behaviour.

Premenstrual Syndrome (PMS)

This is a condition in women that is characterised by emotional and physical symptoms that appear 7 to 14 days before menstruation. These symptoms seem to be related to a hormonal imbalance, of which hypoglycaemia is a common contributing factor.

Migraine headaches

Several medical studies have implicated hypoglycaemia as a common precipitating factor in migraine headaches.

Attention Deficit/Hyperactivity Disorder (ADHD)

A major contributor to the current epidemic of learning and behavioural disorders in our children is the fluctuations in their blood sugar levels.

PREVENTION AND TREATMENT

This common problem can be prevented and treated through lifestyle changes and by avoiding the predisposing factors discussed earlier.

Diet

Eat small frequent meals. Avoid simple carbohydrates and emphasise the adequate intake of healthy proteins and vegetables. A dietary plan called ShapeWorks, developed for Herbalife International by Dr David Heber from UCLA School of Medicine, is an excellent way to correct this problem.

Supplements

The B vitamins, the omega-3 fatty acids and the minerals chromium, vanadium and magnesium all help to control blood sugar levels.

Stress management

Stress aggravates blood sugar imbalances in many ways, especially by exhausting the adrenal glands. The adrenal glands are chiefly responsible for regulating the stress response through the production of stress hormones, like cortisol and adrenaline. Chronic stress can lead to 'adrenal burnout', a condition in which the individual can no longer effectively respond to stress. Adequate rest and relaxation is, therefore, essential.

 Your health is in your hands and so is control over your blood sugar levels.

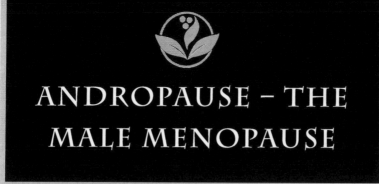

ANDROPAUSE – THE MALE MENOPAUSE

Andropause is the male counterpart to the female menopause. While it is not as rapid, as obvious or as extreme an event as menopause, men do suffer from declining hormone levels as they age.

During menopause, when women are in their fifties, their sex hormones rapidly decline over several years. The sex hormones in men also decline as they age, starting earlier and occurring much more gradually. As one doctor stated, 'women fall off a cliff' while 'men sort of roll down the hill'.

TESTOSTERONE – THE MALE HORMONE

Several hormones, known as androgens, create and support masculinity, but testosterone is the one that is primarily responsible for:

- determining before birth whether a baby will develop male or female features

- influencing an individual's sexual preference

- regulating the sex drive in men and in women* (of course, women do produce small amounts of testosterone, in much the same way that men produce female hormones. It is the balance that is important – the ratio between the male and female hormones – in determining optimal health)

- the development of male physical characteristics including physical strength, emotional assertiveness, body shape, hairiness, a deep voice, and even body odour

- governing the production and quality of sperm.

Additionally, testosterone plays a role in developing creativity, intellect, thought patterns, assertiveness and drive, as well as the ability to produce new ideas and successfully carry them through. It also affects general health during childhood, adolescence and adulthood.

After the age of 30, a man may lose up to two per cent of the function of his testicles (where testosterone is produced) with each succeeding year. In fact, up to 50 per cent of otherwise healthy men between the ages of 50 and 70 have low levels of testosterone.

SIGNS OF ANDROPAUSE

In addition to experiencing a decrease in sexual desire and erectile function, men with a lowered testosterone level may also notice changes in mood and emotions, a decrease in body mass and strength due to loss of muscle tissue, and an increase in body fat. How would you or your male partner answer the following questions?

ADAM (**A**ndrogen **D**eficiency in the **A**geing **M**ale) **Questionnair**e

1.	Do you have a decrease in libido (sex drive)?	Yes	No
2.	Do you have a lack of energy?	Yes	No
3.	Do you have a decrease in strength and/or endurance?	Yes	No
4.	Have you lost height?	Yes	No
5.	Have you noticed a decreased 'enjoyment of life'?	Yes	No
6.	Are you sad and/or grumpy?	Yes	No
7.	Are your erections weaker?	Yes	No
8.	Have you noticed a recent deterioration in your ability to play sports?	Yes	No
9.	Are you falling asleep after dinner?	Yes	No
10.	Has there been a recent deterioration in your work performance?	Yes	No

Answer the questionnaire above. If you answered 'yes' to five or more questions, then you are likely experiencing andropause.

There are also additional health risks associated with low testosterone levels. These include:

- Elevated cholesterol levels
- Heart disease
- Bone fractures
- Clinical depression

HORMONE REPLACEMENT THERAPY

Hormone replacement therapy (HRT) is a powerful intervention in handling andropause as it often produces a significant and dramatic improvement in the symptoms and a reduction in the risks. It involves giving back to the body the hormones that are low, thus restoring normal levels. HRT should be undertaken in a scientific manner following some basic principles:

Test first

Each individual should be medically evaluated and should undergo a simple blood test to measure the levels of testosterone. I particularly recommend doing a special blood test that measures 'free' testosterone in the body. You should also test the levels of other hormones in the blood (such as oestrogen, DHEA – another hormone the body uses to make testosterone, progesterone and thyroid hormones). This is necessary because individual hormones act like instruments in an orchestra. Each one affects the other, and one hormone can often be converted into another. The overall result depends on the balance between all of them. The best results come from checking several different hormones (doing a hormonal profile) and supplementing accordingly.

Use bio-identical hormones

If hormone levels are low, correct them by administering the right dosages of the specific hormone that is deficient in the body, and not with some synthetic drug. This is called bio-identical hormone replacement. If the levels of free testosterone are low, consider having testosterone replacement with a testosterone skin gel. If DHEA is also low, then tablets of DHEA can be taken. If oestrogen or progesterone are imbalanced, this should be corrected also with bio-identical hormones as should any thyroid imbalance.

Monitor

Periodically repeat the blood test and, if necessary, adjust the dosage of the testosterone gel being given to achieve the desired result. If these guidelines are followed, then HRT is an extremely safe and effective anti-aging therapy.

ACTION PLAN

For the man who is concerned about andropause, here are some additional suggestions.

- Consume a healthy diet with enough healthy proteins
- Exercise regularly and pay attention to effective stress management
- Add antioxidants and herbal supplements to your diet, such as the ginsengs, saw palmetto, pygeum africanum, St John's Wort, and pumpkin seed
- Detoxify the body and avoid exposure to toxins and harmful chemicals.

As with menopause, andropause does not have to be the beginning of the end, but rather the passage to a more passionate, purposeful and rewarding time of a man's life.

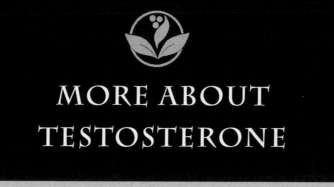

MORE ABOUT
TESTOSTERONE

In the previous chapter, 'Andropause – The Male Menopause', I introduced the major male hormone, testosterone, and emphasised the importance of maintaining optimal levels of this hormone as we age. A nutritional and dietary program was outlined that can be very helpful in that regard. Now we will consider other lifestyle issues that influence the testosterone levels of both men and women.

EXERCISE

Both a lack of physical activity as well as an excess of physical activity will result in decreased levels of testosterone. Exercise affects testosterone directly by stimulating the pituitary gland (in the brain) as well as the testicles. The duration, frequency and intensity of the exercise will determine the levels of testosterone in the bloodstream.

Testosterone levels increase most with short, intense bursts of activity (like strength training and weight lifting), and decrease with prolonged endurance activities, such as long distance running, swimming or cycling. During endurance training, testosterone is needed to maintain muscle integrity, but frequent extended training does not allow for repair and recovery and tissue damage may occur. Studies show that short intensive exercise will elevate testosterone for about 45 minutes, but if prolonged for over an hour the effects become negative and the levels begin to fall. Once they are down, they stay down for as long as six days.

To maximise your testosterone response to exercise and to avoid overtraining, follow these guidelines:

- Do strength training (weight lifting/resistance exercises) for no more than 45 minutes, three to four times per week. Alternate that with endurance/fitness type exercises.

- If you want to exercise or train more, split sessions are recommended, for example, weight training in the morning and aerobic training in the evening.

- Allow adequate time for your muscles to recover between workouts. Exercise different muscles on consecutive training days.

- Follow the nutritional guidelines previously outlined.

ALCOHOL USE

Reduce or eliminate alcohol use. Excessive drinking can increase the levels of female hormones and inhibit the body's ability to produce testosterone. By not drinking alcohol, you allow your liver to better remove excessive female hormones from the body.

MEDICATION

Eliminate all medications that are unnecessary for your health. Many commonly prescribed drugs affect liver function and testosterone conversion. This list includes the anti-inflammatory drugs like ibuprofen, acetaminophen, aspirin and the 'statin' class of cholesterol lowering drugs, some heart and blood pressure lowering medication and some antidepressants.

Consult with your physician and ask if the medications can be stopped for a six-month period so as to determine how they may be affecting your hormonal levels. Many of these 'lifestyle medications' may be actually treating the symptoms of testosterone deficiency, and you may no longer need them after following the approaches we have been discussing.

REST AND SUNSHINE

Try to get as close to eight hours of sleep nightly. Studies have shown that most of us are chronically sleep deprived, and nothing can take the place of adequate rest. If you are sleep deprived, your testosterone status will suffer. If you cannot get that many hours of sleep regularly, try having power naps during the day.

Aim to have some direct exposure to sunlight daily. Try being outdoors for at least one hour daily. Testosterone rises and falls with the seasons, and sunrise is necessary for healthy body rhythms and optimal testosterone production.

STRESS MANAGEMENT

There is a strong relationship between mental outlook and physical wellness, and this is largely mediated by hormones. This right kind of stress can have a positive impact on our hormones, but the wrong kind of chronic stress can be devastating. Ongoing emotional stress and depression are common causes of decreased testosterone levels, leading to premature ageing. Learn stress management techniques.

HORMONE REPLACEMENT THERAPY

Hormone replacement therapy is, in my opinion, just as important in men as in women. I use bio-identical hormones in the form of trans-dermal testosterone skin creams. I also recommend the use of pro-hormones – substances that the body itself will convert into testosterone, using the body's own checks and balances, and minimising potential unwanted side effects.

This kind of treatment should be supervised by a health care professional who is experienced in using these methods. So, gentlemen, adopt a testosterone enhancing lifestyle and enjoy the benefits.

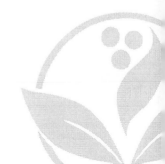

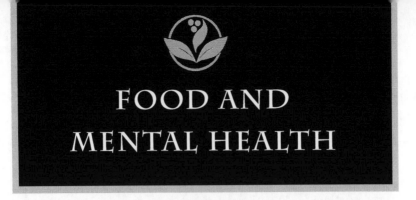

FOOD AND MENTAL HEALTH

Research by the Mental Health Foundation in the United Kingdom suggests that the modern diet has altered the balance of certain key nutrients in our food and is affecting our mental health.

They say that not eating enough fresh food and consuming too many processed foods loaded with unhealthy fats and sugars are leading to depression, anxiety, memory problems and other mental disorders. Food experts claim the research is not conclusive, but doctors in Canada have treated thousands of patients with a variety of mental illnesses with a nutritional approach called Orthomolecular Psychiatry. They have successfully used food and vitamins to treat major psychiatric disorders.

Let us look at how food can affect the way your brain functions.

ESSENTIAL FATTY ACID IMBALANCE

Sixty per cent of the dry weight of the brain is comprised of fat, particularly essential fatty acids (EFAs) like omega-3s. These are good fats which, unfortunately, are not readily provided in the Jamaican diet. EFAs are important components of nerve cell walls and are involved in the transmission of electrical activity in the brain.

Lack of these fats can cause the brain to malfunction and promote mental illness. For example, nerve cell degeneration and brain shrinkage are commonly found among people with chronic schizophrenia. They show an increased breakdown of the walls of nerve cells in certain areas of the brain. For sufferers of schizophrenia and other mental illnesses, such as Attention Deficit Hyperactivity Disorder (ADHD) and depression, omega-3 fats offer a means of maintaining brain membrane structure and avoiding brain mass loss. Several major medical centres around the world are now using high doses of omega-3 fats to treat these conditions.

BRAIN ALLERGIES

Like any other organ in the body, the brain can suffer from allergies. Fifteen per cent of people with schizophrenia have brain allergies. Cerebral allergies involve a gut reaction when poorly digested food particles are absorbed into the blood stream – the so-called 'Leaky Gut Syndrome'. This ultimately perpetuates the release of brain toxins that result in psychosis, malaise, depression, irritability, and so on.

Culprit foods and culprit environmental compounds can account for some cases of schizophrenia. An investigative test called an elimination diet is used for diagnosing this problem. Individualised nutritional programs can be essential in the management of schizophrenia.

Testing for overgrowth of gut organisms, like yeast, as well as for other toxic by-products may also be necessary when cerebral allergies are suspected.

SUGAR IMBALANCE

The main fuel on which the brain runs is glucose – the sugar found in the blood. Imbalance in blood sugar levels can lead to brain dysfunction. Hypoglycaemia is the term that describes low sugar in the blood. Irritability, poor memory, poor concentration, tiredness, cold hands, muscle cramping, sugar cravings and 'feeling temporarily better then worse after eating carbohydrates' are typical hypoglycaemic symptoms.

Hypoglycaemia tends to be an aggravating factor in mental illnesses since the brain cells are being starved of fuel. The nutritional treatment for hypoglycaemia involves dietary changes and supplements. Hypoglycaemia is one hundred per cent correctable in patients willing to adhere to the diet.

VITAMIN AND MINERAL DEFICIENCY

Many vitamins and minerals are essential for normal brain function. For example, niacin (vitamin B_3) can affect the metabolism of adrenaline in the brain. This may be a causative factor in schizophrenia or Parkinson's disease.

This biochemical theory was the first presented in the medical literature by Canadian psychiatrists Dr Abram Hoffer and Dr Humphry Osmond and is called the adrenochrome hypothesis. Niacin also plays a role in the essential fatty acid metabolism of the brain that is disrupted in schizophrenia. Niacin, along with vitamin C, is active in the brain creating a calming effect.

Vitamin B_{12}, folic acid and other B vitamins, magnesium, chromium and zinc are a few of the other nutrients that affect brain function.

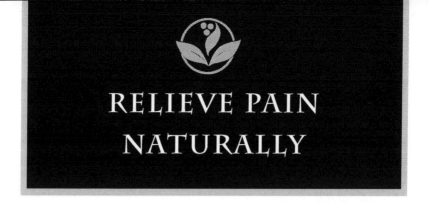

RELIEVE PAIN NATURALLY

'Pain is inevitable; suffering is optional.'

The shelves in your local pharmacy are lined with a bewildering array of drugs for the relief of pain. Many of them are available without a doctor's prescription. They include well-known drugs like aspirin and acetaminophen, as well as a large group of pain relievers called NSAIDs (Non-Steroidal Anti-Inflammatory Drugs) which include Advil, Brufen, Indomethacin and Voltaren.

DRAWBACKS OF PAINKILLERS

These medicines are widely used, often abused and, contrary to popular belief, are far from harmless. Let me share with you some facts about some of them.

ASPIRIN

The chemical name for aspirin is acetylsalicylic acid (ASA). It was first made in 1853 and has since become a preferred treatment for arthritis pain, headaches and fever. Today, many people reach for this drug at the first hint of pain and many doctors recommend that it be taken on a daily basis for the prevention of heart attacks, the commonest killer today. It could be considered the most popular drug in history.

Aspirin is a drug generally regarded as being safe enough to not require a prescription. A normal dose of aspirin for pain is two tablets every four to six hours per day, but an arthritis sufferer might be told by the doctor to take more than twice this amount.

Unfortunately, aspirin has serious side effects. Just look at this list: gastritis, peptic ulcer, intestinal bleeding, haemorrhagic shock, and even sudden death. Aspirin can also affect your eyes by increasing the risk of macular degeneration, a leading cause of blindness. There is even up to a 500 per cent increase in the risk of cataracts among individuals below age 55, who have been taking aspirin over the long term. Aspirin is also one of the leading causes of death from poisoning each year.

ACETAMINOPHEN

Over a third of Americans (and many Jamaicans) take acetaminophen (for example, Tylenol) at least once a month, making it the most widely used pain reliever in the United States. Taking more than the recommended dose, however, can lead to fatal liver injury. Acetaminophen poisoning is now the most common cause of acute liver failure in the United States. Attempted suicides account for many cases, but almost half are the result of unintentional overdoses. And those who had unintentionally taken overdoses usually have even worse outcomes than those who have done so intentionally, since unintentional overdoses are usually not recognised as such immediately.

NSAIDs

As more people develop chronic pain, the drug companies churn out more and more of this class of painkiller. With chronic use, these drugs create many problems like gastritis, bleeding peptic ulcers and kidney damage, as well as increased destruction of cartilage in arthritic joints. Yet, many people are kept on these medications for decades.

Pain is an important clue that your body gives you and it is usually trying to warn you to correct the underlying disorder. Pain is a symptom, not a disease. The best and foremost action you can take is to seek to identify the cause of your pain. Then, even if you need to take something for pain relief, you can also begin to deal with the underlying cause.

NATURAL AND SAFE PAIN RELIEVERS

Fish oils

The omega-3 fatty acids EPA and DHA found in fish oil have been shown, by many clinical studies, to have powerful anti-inflammatory properties that reduce inflammation and promote joint lubrication.

Ginger

This root is anti-inflammatory and offers pain relief and stomach-settling properties. Fresh ginger works well when steeped in boiling water as a tea or grated into vegetable juice. It may also be applied externally as a pack to painful joints and muscles.

Boswellia

This herb contains specific active anti-inflammatory ingredients known as boswellic acids that research has shown significantly reduce inflammation.

Bromelain

This enzyme, found in pineapples, is a natural anti-inflammatory. It can be taken in supplement form, but eating fresh pineapple may also be helpful.

Cayenne cream

Also called capsaicin cream, this spice comes from dried hot peppers. It alleviates pain by depleting the body's supply of substance P, a chemical component of nerve cells that transmits pain signals to the brain.

Aromatherapy

Essential oils like lavender and rosemary offer powerful stress-relieving and analgesic properties. Simply rub a few drops of the oil in your palms and inhale the fragrance for a few moments and notice the change in your feelings.

Energy therapies

Pain responds well to a variety of therapies like hypnosis, acupuncture, emotional freedom therapy and therapeutic touch. The wonderful thing is that many of these treatments can be self-administered.

Before taking two pain pills, consider your options. There are often safer, gentler ways.

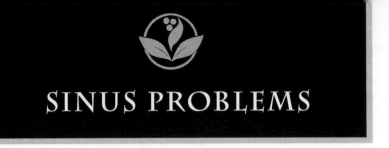

SINUS PROBLEMS

A common Jamaican complaint is 'I have sinus', meaning 'I am having problems with my sinuses'. What is a sinus? In medicine, a sinus is a sac or a cavity in any organ or tissue.

The human skull contains four major pairs of hollow, air-filled cavities called sinuses. These are connected to the nostrils and the nasal passages. The sinuses reduce the weight of the skull and allow the voice to resonate within it. Perhaps most importantly, the sinuses provide defences against harmful foreign substances in the air like germs, dust, smoke, particles in the air and chemical pollutants. It should come as no surprise that, as the air we breathe and the environment we live in become more polluted, more of our people complain of sinus problems. Sinusitis is simply an inflammation of the membranes lining the sinuses.

Sinusitis is one of the leading chronic diseases and, according to the American Academy of Otolaryngology, over 37 million Americans have one or more episodes of sinusitis a year. These are caused by allergies or colds, which inflame the sinuses. Americans lose more than 73 million days from work and school each year when they stay home due to sinusitis. I wonder about the situation in Jamaica!

SYMPTOMS OF SINUSITIS

Common symptoms include facial pain or pressure, nasal obstruction, nasal discharge, diminished sense of smell, irritation of the throat, drainage and cough. Additionally, sufferers may have fever, bad breath, fatigue and even dental pain.

TREATMENT

Sadly, modern medicine focuses its attention on treating the symptoms of this problem with drugs and surgery. Virtually no attention is paid to treating the underlying causes or on prevention. I know patients who have been on 'sinus medication' for over 20 years! Many of these people have rapidly learned how to get rid of the problem or greatly improve it.

A natural approach

- **Clean up your diet.**

Unburden your system of chemicals and food additives. Minimise your intake of processed foods, including sugar and white flour. Most importantly, take a holiday from all dairy products – cow's milk, butter, cheese, ice cream and so on. Dairy products stimulate mucus production from the sinuses. Read food labels carefully. Consume lots of fresh fruits and vegetables and drink more water.

- **Clean up your environment.**

Do all you can to avoid pollutants in your surroundings, such as mould, dust, pollen and chemicals which are found in the air you breathe. Avoid damp, poorly ventilated areas and rid curtains, mats, pillows, pets and toys of allergens. Be aware that paint, new carpets and furniture will emit toxic chemicals for a long time. Avoid cigarette smoke.

- **Strengthen your immune system.**

Take lots of antioxidants. These include the ACES – vitamins A, C and E and the mineral selenium. Also, boost your intake of herbs and other nutrients.

I particularly recommend a combination of the herbs schizandra and rosemary along with the ACES. These are conveniently available and can be found mixed together in tablet form.

- **Wash and humidify your sinuses.**

For thousands of years, practitioners of yoga have used a technique called neti to keep their sinuses and nostrils in excellent condition. This was particularly important to them as they considered good breathing essential to good health.

I use this method myself and strongly recommend it to sinus sufferers as well as to anyone interested in excellent health. It involves the use of a simple and inexpensive device called a *neti* pot that looks like a small teapot. The pot is filled with warm salt (natural salt, such as sea salt) water and the spout applied to a nostril. By tilting the head back, you can allow the water to run into one nostril and out of the other nostril. The method is easy to use and learn. A few dos and don'ts are easily understood. Daily use of this technique cleanses and humidifies the nasal passages and not only relieves sinus symptoms but also prevents future attacks.

In my experience, this simple holistic approach designed to have your own body do the healing and prevention of sinusitis is an excellent method. It allows you to avoid many of the dangers and problems of drugs and surgery. Of course, these traditional treatments may have their place but, should, in my opinion, be reserved for special, acute situations or when these simple methods have not been effective enough.

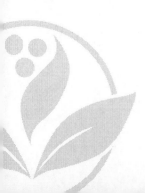

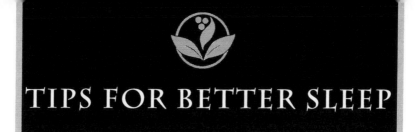

TIPS FOR BETTER SLEEP

Research shows that sleep problems affect about 35 per cent of the population. But in certain groups like menopausal women the incidence may be as high as 75 per cent. Most adults will experience some type of sleep problem in their lifetime without any major inconvenience, but if the loss of quality sleep continues for long it can have negative effects.

Insomnia is usually a symptom of an underlying problem and not a disease in itself. Stress, depression, illness, medication or poor diet may be the underlying causes. The actual amount of sleep we need varies from person to person. Some people can do quite well with less than five hours of sleep, while others may need as many as ten or more hours of sleep. A sleep deficit of only a few hours can result in irritability, fatigue and poor concentration, and can affect our ability to stay alert during the day.

As we get older, changes occur in our sleep patterns and there is a tendency for our sleep to begin and end earlier. The quality of our sleep also changes. Less time is spent in the deeper forms of sleep and so our sleep is more easily interrupted by noise, the need to take a trip to the bathroom, or physical discomfort. The problem is further compounded, as falling back to sleep becomes harder to do.

Sleep is essential to life and the quality and quantity of sleep is critical to good health. If you have been experiencing some sleepless nights, here are some suggestions to help improve your chances of a better night's sleep. If your sleep problems persist for longer than a couple of weeks, you should discuss it with your physician or medical practitioner.

AVOID HUNGER OR OVEREATING AT BEDTIME

Eating increases the heart rate, which makes it difficult to sleep, while a full stomach increases the risk of acid reflux and heartburn. On the other hand, the discomfort of hunger can keep you awake especially if your blood sugar gets low. Try having a light snack a couple of hours before bedtime.

STOP SMOKING

The nicotine in tobacco smoke is an even stronger stimulant than caffeine. Research shows that smokers tend to take longer to fall asleep and often wake up during the night with cravings for nicotine. By the way, smoking in bed is even more dangerous.

CUT BACK ON PM DRINKS

A full bladder can wake you and, once awake, you might experience trouble falling back to sleep. Alcohol and caffeine both adversely affect sleep and increase the frequency of urination. Even though alcohol may help you temporarily go to sleep, it will disrupt the pattern and quality of your night's sleep.

DEVELOP REGULAR PATTERNS

Regularly going to bed and getting up at the same time every day helps keep your biological clock in rhythm. This influences your body's production of key hormones like melatonin and cortisol, which are substances that powerfully influence your sleep patterns.

UNWIND BEFORE BEDTIME

Read, listen to music, or watch a relaxing television program for about half an hour before bedtime. Take a warm bath, making it special with candles and bath oils.

MAKE YOUR BEDROOM SLEEP FRIENDLY

Keep work and other activities out of the bedroom. Television and computers can become sleep robbers. Draperies or blinds can reduce noise and the morning light. If you find yourself unable to go to sleep, do not toss around in bed. Get up and read, listen to instrumental music or meditate until you become sleepy once again.

CHOOSE THE RIGHT BED

Invest in a good mattress and pillows. They should not be too firm or too soft. The better beds adjust to your body's contours while still providing optimal support.

EXERCISE REGULARLY

Being fit helps to make you more resistant to the stresses that can keep you awake at night. Research shows that active people tend to rest better. But, you should avoid vigorous activity within two hours of bedtime as this stimulation may keep you awake. The exception to this is sex, which most people report actually helps them fall asleep.

USE NATURAL SLEEP AIDS

Valerian, kava, chamomile, Tang Kuei, St John's Wort, lavender oil and melatonin are all good natural sleep aids, which do not have the harmful side effects of sleeping tablets. These can be used in combination with the strategies mentioned above. The relaxation and breathing exercises presented on my CD, *A Time to Relax*, are also excellent tools to improve the quality of your sleep.

 Make your sleep natural, healthy and restful.

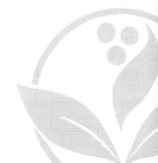

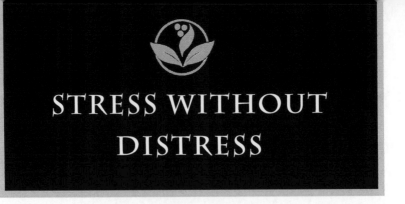

STRESS WITHOUT DISTRESS

'Tension is who you think you should be.
Relaxation is who you are.'
– Chinese Proverb

It seems that in every period in his history, man has been subjected to some form of deadly threat or disease. Today, perhaps the greatest challenge to health is not heart disease or cancer or diabetes or AIDS. No, I believe that the greatest threat that we face is stress. Stress underlies much of our suffering.

Stress contributes to such a very long list of disorders, some of them life threatening, that researchers at Cornell University Medical College in New York called stress 'the most debilitating medical condition in the United States'. Sadly, we spend a great deal of time and money treating these symptoms while failing to recognise and address the underlying cause – STRESS!

The word stress is the current buzz word. Everyone complains about it and blames it for everything, from flu and headaches to high blood pressure and cancer. Some authorities claim that 70 to 80 per cent of the patients who visit the doctor are suffering from stress-related disorders. It is hard to imagine how a single entity can produce so many problems.

WHAT IS STRESS?

It is extremely important to understand that stress is not a thing, it is a response! Stress is the internal response that an individual has to an external stimulus. We humans are very good at finding scapegoats to blame for the way we feel. I am sorry, but stress is not your spouse or your financial situation. It is not what is happening on the outside. It is how you choose to respond internally to those external instigating factors. The external events are called stressors while your internal reaction is the stress. The enemy is within.

Understanding the simple distinction between stress and stressor is crucial to effective stress management. Very often, we cannot change the external factors (stressors), but we can learn to control our internal response to those stressors. We don't have to be victims. We have the power and the ability to choose. The most powerful source of stress is in our own minds.

HOW DOES STRESS AFFECT US?

Science is becoming more and more aware of how powerfully the mind and its thoughts affect the body. Common manifestations of stress are:

- Sleep disorders

- Anxiety and nervousness

- Headaches, dizziness and various unusual sensations in the head

- Sexual problems such as impotence or low libido

- Digestive problems such as gas, diarrhoea or constipation and Irritable Bowel Syndrome

- Depression, low energy, emotional and mental disturbances, and difficulty concentrating

- Ringing in the ears, chest pain and backache

- Awareness of heartbeat and difficulty in breathing

- Tingling or numbness in the hands and/or feet

- High blood pressure

- Menstrual disturbance, infertility and hormone imbalances

- Accident proneness and phobias

- Poor performance, for example, in examinations

It is important to realise that stress is not necessarily a bad thing. Life will always have its stressors. If we can handle them well, they can serve to stimulate us to greater strength and accomplishments.

Good stress management is not simply trying to avoid stressors; that may not be possible or even advisable. The idea is to learn how to handle and deal with stressors effectively. In the same way that the body has a stress reaction, the 'fight or flight' response, so too is there also a relaxation response. This occurs when the body calms and releases its tension and the brain produces its own tranquilizers (endorphins) in the right amount at the right time and without side effects. Learning how to elicit this relaxation response is the key to good stress management.

HOW TO MANAGE STRESS

There are several tools and techniques that can help you to deal with stress effectively. Some of these are listed here.

- Identify and list your main stressors. Become aware of your reactions to them. Learn to observe yourself in stressful situations so you can begin to choose how you respond instead of having an unconscious reaction. Don't react. Respond.

- Explore ways to elicit your relaxation response. Different people have different activities that relax them, for example, listening to music, engaging in your favourite hobby, social work, and so on. I particularly recommend the audio CD program, *A Time to Relax*. It contains specially composed music by my colleague Dr Winsome Miller-Rowe, while I lead you through a series of breathing and visualisation exercises designed to teach you how to put yourself into deep relaxation. It is particularly helpful for people who have difficulty falling asleep.

- Daily exercise, particularly yoga, deep breathing, meditation, self hypnosis and visualisation exercises are most beneficial.

- Seek professional help for counselling or psychotherapy if necessary. This helps you to identify the underlying source of your stress and to develop better ways of releasing it.

- Be extremely careful about using drugs to alleviate symptoms of stress. This includes recreational drugs like alcohol and marijuana as well as prescription medicines like Valium and Ativan. They only give temporary relief and are all addictive.

- A proper diet is extremely important. Aim to include five or more servings of fresh fruit and vegetables daily along with an optimal protein intake. I recommend the Cellular Nutrition Program with nutritional supplements like fish oils with omega-3 fats, magnesium and the B vitamins.

Avoid sugar, artificial sweeteners, MSG, hydrogenated oils and fried foods.

- The herbs Tang Kuei, chamomile, kava, St John's Wort and valerian are excellent non-drug alternatives to tranquiliser medication. The advice of a qualified health care professional on the choice, combinations and use of these herbs is important, especially in individuals with significant anxiety and/or depression.

I teach a special yoga technique called Yoga Nidra that is a particularly useful tool in stress management.

STROKE RECOVERY

*'So many people spend their health gaining wealth, and then have
to spend their wealth to regain their health.'*
– A.J. Reb Materi

In a previous article I outline a program for preventing strokes. Unfortunately, many have not avoided this medical disaster. Stroke continues to be the third most frequent cause of death in the western world. Of those who survive a stroke, only 10 per cent are able to return to their work without disability. The United States spends $30 billion annually caring for stroke victims, and the emotional cost to patients, their families and their caregivers is incalculable.

Until recently, the medical dogma was that there was essentially no chance of any further meaningful recovery from a stroke after the first few months following the event. New scientific research reveals that this pessimistic view, still held by many doctors, is clearly unwarranted.

When a stroke occurs, cells in an area of the brain die. There is also an adjacent area where other brain cells are damaged and dysfunctional but not dead. These cells are functional but not functioning and can remain in this state of idling for a long time. They are like cars parked with their motors running, waiting to be put into gear. Strategies are available that can revive these damaged cells even if the stroke occurred years ago.

5-STEP STROKE RECOVERY PROGRAM

Here is a 5-step stroke recovery program.

Step 1: Nutrition

Optimal nutrition is vital, as it is by providing the body with the right combination of nutrients at a cellular level that you can stimulate the body's amazing healing capacity. I use and recommend a plan called the Cellular Nutrition Program along with guidelines for healthy eating.

Step 2: Supplement

There are specific additional nutritional supplements that facilitate brain repair:

- Vitamins B_6, B_{12}, folic acid, vitamins E and C. These are essential for the metabolism of the brain cells, for preventing free radical damage and improving the circulation.

- Coenzyme Q10, and NADH (Nicotinamide Adenide Dinucleotide). These natural substances increase the energy levels in damaged brain cells and facilitate healing. They are available in health food stores.

- Phosphatidylserene (PS) is a key component of healthy brain cells. It facilitates energy production in the cells of the brain as well as cell to cell communication.

- Fish oils. They contain omega-3 fatty acids and are very effective in controlling the inflammatory reactions in brain cells that occur when they are damaged.

Step 3: Herbs

- **Vinpocetine.** This is an extract of the lesser periwinkle plant, Vinca minor. It has been proven to improve the clinical outcome of stroke patients and has been widely used in over 35 countries around the world. It increases blood flow to the brain, is a powerful antioxidant and prevents blood cells from clumping together, thus further improving the circulation.

- **Ginkgo biloba.** This herb has a long history of use in China and is now extensively utilised in European medicine for the treatment of a variety of brain disorders. It improves the cerebral metabolism and circulation while acting as an antioxidant.

Step 4: Hyperbaric oxygen therapy

Hyperbaric oxygen therapy (HBOT) is a truly exciting medical treatment that I was first exposed to on a visit to Cuba many years ago. There, HBOT is widely used in all hospitals for a variety of conditions including strokes. This treatment involves exposing the patient to pure oxygen under increased atmospheric pressure. This enhances the levels of oxygen in the tissues even in areas where the circulation is poor or absent and cellular damage exists. The oxygen facilitates the growth of new blood vessels and increases cellular repair and healing. I consider it a serious indictment of our health care system that not one of our hospitals in Jamaica offers hyperbaric oxygen therapy. This technology has many uses, is extremely cost effective and readily available. Right now I recommend that you go to Cuba or Florida if you need it.

Step 5: Physical therapy

The experts agree that the treatments outlined above work best when combined with physical, occupational and speech therapy. These should be aggressively pursued on an ongoing basis. Fortunately, excellent therapists offer these treatments here in Jamaica.

**Please understand, IT IS NEVER TOO LATE.
You or your loved ones can begin a stroke
recovery program right now!**

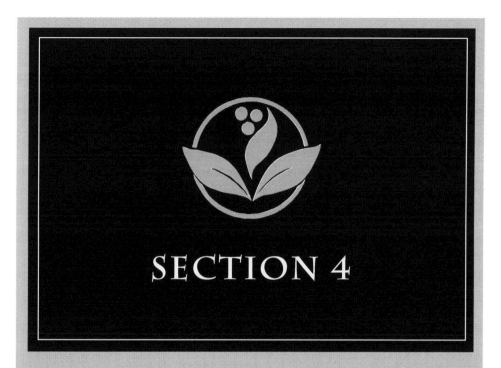

SECTION 4

FEMALE
ISSUES

'As I see it, every day you do one of two things: build health or produce disease in yourself.'

– Adelle Davis, noted female Natural Health Advocate

www.anounceofprevention.org

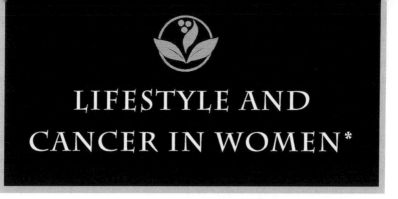

LIFESTYLE AND
CANCER IN WOMEN*

Recent medical research indicates that a woman's risk of developing cancer is largely under her control. It's all about choices. If you make the lifestyle choices that promote cancer, you'll probably get cancer. If you make informed, healthy choices, you are much more likely to avoid this deadly disease.

Amazingly, many people, even some doctors, still don't acknowledge the huge connection between lifestyle choices and chronic diseases like cancer. Some still believe disease is just a matter of chance, or that it's entirely determined by your genes. That's not true. Your level of health is, to a very great extent, under your own control.

Post-menopausal women, in particular, who follow recommended dietary and lifestyle guidelines may significantly reduce their risk of developing and dying from cancer, according to recent research.

Dr James Cerhan at the Mayo Clinic in the US had reported on research involving almost 30,000 women, aged over 55 years. Dr Cerhan's team evaluated these women's risk of cancer based on how many healthy lifestyle habits they practised. These habits were the ones recommended by the American Association for Cancer Research.

Those women who followed one or none of the recommended guidelines for diet and lifestyle had a 35 per cent higher risk of developing cancer and a 42 per cent greater risk of dying from cancer than women who adhered to most of the recommendations considered in the study.

Those recommendations developed by the American Association for Cancer Research are as follows:

- Engage in daily moderate exercise and vigorous physical activity at least once per week.

- Maintain normal body weight and/or keep your weight within ten pounds of the weight you were at age 18.

- Eat five or more servings of vegetables and fruit daily.

- Limit your red meat consumption to less than three ounces per day.

- Limit your daily consumption of unhealthy animal fats.

- Limit your alcohol intake to no more than one drink per day.

- Refrain from cigarette smoking.

In short, the research shows that older women may reduce their risk of dying from cancer by almost half by simply not smoking, controlling body weight, exercising and eating a healthy, balanced diet.

Dr Joseph Mercola, a noted wellness expert, suggests that this study barely scratches the surface of what's really possible. If Dr Cerhan and his team had studied women who do *everything right* – that is, who avoid all processed foods, who follow a Cellular Nutrition Program, who eat whole foods, who avoid cancer-causing ingredients like sodium nitrite, aspartame and MSG, who avoid artificial harmful chemicals in their personal care products, and who take other similar precautions – they'd find the cancer rate approaching ZERO. Cancer doesn't need to exist at all. It actually should be a rarity except for that fact that most women actually *give themselves cancer* by making poor choices in life.

It is now estimated that one in three women will develop cancer during her lifetime. It is, therefore, important that we, as a society, spend so much more effort, time and money on preventing cancer.

---

*Although I focus on women in this chapter, the content applies to men as well.

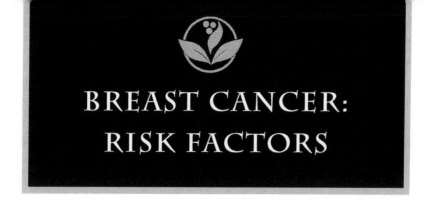

BREAST CANCER: RISK FACTORS

Breast cancer statistics over the years

1950 – 1 in 20 women had breast cancer
1970 – 1 in 14 women had breast cancer
2000 – 1 in 8 women had breast cancer
2020 – ? ? ?

Despite all the emphasis on the early detection of breast cancer with annual campaigns and rousing slogans, the incidence of this deadly disease continues to rise at an alarming rate – over 60 per cent in the last 60 years.

It is therefore clear that the old approach is not working. Most of our resources are spent on early detection. I believe that if the special interest groups like the Ministry of Health and the Jamaica Cancer Society put more effort into really promoting prevention, rather than just early detection, more could be accomplished. **Breast cancer can be prevented!**

WHAT CAUSES BREAST CANCER?

The evidence is overwhelming that the female sex hormone, oestrogen, is closely connected to the development of most cases of breast cancer. Oestrogen encourages the tissue cells in the breast to multiply more rapidly. It is the oestrogen-dependent type of breast cancer that is the most common type today.

The average woman in today's world is exposed to more oestrogen than ever before, especially to unhealthier or 'bad' forms of oestrogen. This puts our women at serious risk. The following are some risk factors for breast cancer that are not often emphasised. They may be divided into three categories.

Medical risk factors

1. Oral contraceptives, especially with early and prolonged use.

2. Oestrogen replacement therapy (commonly used in menopausal women), especially with high doses and prolonged use.

3. Early and repeated exposure to mammograms before menopause. The National Cancer Institute in the US released evidence that, among women under 35, mammography could cause 75 cases of breast cancer for every 15 cases it identifies.

4. Silicone breast implants, especially those using polyurethane foam.

5. Certain non-hormonal prescription drugs such as some hypertension medicines, antibiotics, tranquilisers, antidepressants, cholesterol lowering drugs, and the very drugs used to treat cancer itself. Yes, patients on chemotherapy drugs for cancer have an increased risk of developing another type of cancer.

Dietary and environmental risk factors

1. A diet high in animal fat (beef, poultry and dairy products) contaminated with undisclosed cancer-causing and oestrogen-like chemicals.

2. Exposure in the home to household chemicals such as cleansers, aerosols and pesticides, or pollution from neighbouring chemical plants.

3. Exposure at the workplace to a wide variety of cancer-causing chemicals.

Lifestyle risk factors

1. Alcohol, especially with early and excessive use.

2. Tobacco, especially with early and excessive use.

3. Inactivity, obesity and a sedentary lifestyle.

4. Dark hair dyes, with early and prolonged use.

5. Prolonged stress, when inadequately managed.

The onus is on every woman to make a serious commitment to avoid these factors that are known to put them at risk for developing breast cancer. The really sad thing is that the factors listed above relate not only to breast cancer but also to fibrocystic disease of the breast, uterine fibroids, premenstrual syndrome (PMS), endometriosis and cancer of the uterus among others. Many of these factors also put our men at risk for prostate cancer and low sperm counts.

 Knowledge is power. Put this knowledge to work for you.

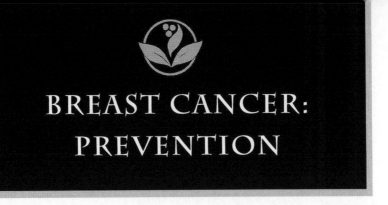

BREAST CANCER: PREVENTION

More people will be diagnosed with breast cancer this year than last year, despite the best efforts of the breast cancer awareness campaigns. The problem is that the focus is on early detection and then treatment of breast cancer, while very little attention is aimed at prevention. After all, diagnosing and treating cancer is a huge and profitable business. Do not expect those powerful business interests to give much attention to preventing what is so profitable to treat.

The health of your breasts is really your concern. You must take responsibility for your own cancer prevention program. Prevention is infinitely better than cure, and breast cancer can be prevented.

5-STEP PREVENTION PLAN

Here is a 5-step plan that you can follow to help you prevent breast cancer.

Step 1: Eat right

- **Eat a diet low in fat and high in fibre.** The major part of your diet should come from plant based foods such as fresh vegetables, fruits, whole grains, whole grain cereals, beans, legumes, ground provisions, vegetable soups and fresh juices. Research shows that the fibre in these foods actually helps the body eliminate cancer-causing oestrogens from the body.

- **Minimise your intake of animal meats and dairy products.** These foods are the major dietary sources of cancer-causing chemicals and dangerous oestrogen-like hormones. The fatty parts of beef, chicken and pork are particularly dangerous as the harmful chemicals are usually fat-soluble and are concentrated in the fatty tissues. Tinned, preserved or fried meats, for example, bacon and sausage, contain the preservative sodium nitrite which is also cancer-causing.

- **Eat soy-based foods.** They contain natural substances called *isoflavones* that protect the breast from cancer. These substances act like very weak hormones and protect the cells in the breast from the powerful chemical hormones.

  Despite any unsubstantiated stories you may hear, there is no medical evidence that soy causes cancer. On the contrary, the research suggests that increased soy consumption decreases the risk of many cancers including breast and prostate cancer. A good soy-based protein shake taken daily is a convenient way to ensure regular soy supplementation. Fermented soy foods like tofu, miso, tempeh and textured vegetable protein are also good. Roasted soy nuts are an excellent anti-cancer snack.

- **Drink green tea.** Japanese research indicates that women who drink two or more cups of green tea daily reduce their risk of breast cancer by 50 per cent.

- **Eat cruciferous vegetables regularly.** These include cabbage, broccoli, cauliflower and Brussels sprouts. Other vegetables such as tomatoes and carrots that contain powerful anti-cancer agents should also be eaten frequently. Emphasise variety and colour in your choice of vegetables.

- **Minimise your intake of sugar.** For many reasons, sugar promotes the growth of cancer cells. The more processed a food, the more chemicals (including sugar) are added to it. Focus on more natural foods with less preservatives and additives.

Step 2: Take supplements

- **Take a good multivitamin and mineral supplement.** I recommend tablets that are taken to supplement each meal on a daily basis. I also recommend the antioxidants, vitamins A, C, E and selenium (the ACES), as well as the antioxidant herbs – schizandra and rosemary.

- **Take melatonin.** This is a hormone produced by the pineal gland in your brain. It is available as a supplement. Artificial lighting reduces our natural production of melatonin and taking it as a supplement has been shown to aid in the prevention and treatment of breast cancer.

- **Take herbs.** Red clover and Kudzu, like soy, contain isoflavones. Black Cohosh and Tang Kuei are herbs that promote a healthy hormonal balance in women. These are conveniently available as tablets or teas. A holistic practitioner can advise you on their use.

Step 3: Change your lifestyle

- **Correct and avoid obesity.** Obesity is a risk factor for breast cancer. Fat cells create additional oestrogen and this can promote breast cancer. Also, fat women discover their breast cancer later than slim women do. Weight (fat) loss along with moderate exercise will decrease your cancer risk and provide several other health benefits.

- **Avoid toxins.** Stay away from tobacco smoke, as it causes cancer. Avoid, or at least minimise, alcohol intake. Drinking alcohol increases the levels of oestrogen in your blood.

- **Be extremely careful with hair dyes.** One study reported that 87 out 100 breast cancer patients had been long-term users of hair dye. Many semi-permanent and permanent hair dyes are a witch's brew of carcinogens. Use safer, natural alternatives for hair care and skin care.

- **Avoid environmental pollution and unnecessary drug use (prescription or otherwise).** Be careful with household chemicals. Follow a regular internal cleansing and detoxification program.

- **Expose your skin to sunshine.** Half an hour in the morning or late afternoon sun is ideal. The darker your skin the more sunshine you need. The sun uses cholesterol in your skin to create vitamin D in the right quantities for your needs. Optimal levels of vitamin D protect against many cancers including breast and prostate cancer. Regular sunshine also improves the body's production of melatonin.

- **Learn to detect and manage stress.** This is very important. Chronic stress causes raised levels of the stress hormone cortisol. High cortisol levels may impair the body's immune system and weaken your resistance to cancer and other diseases.

Step 4: Manage menopause naturally

- **Consider bio-identical hormone replacement therapy.** This is an alternative to synthetic and horse-derived hormones. Hormone replacement can be both safe and effective if we first determine which hormone the body needs and then replace what is missing with the same substance. That is what I mean by bio-identical hormone replacement. Natural progesterone, for example, is available as a skin cream and is a useful tool in managing menopause while protecting the breast from cancer.

Step 5: Check your breasts

While on your prevention program, it is wise to check for any pre-existent breast lumps. Some women are afraid to examine their breasts. Do not give in to your fears. When it comes to breast cancer, ignorance is not bliss. Regular examination of your breasts is essential.

- **Use mammograms very sparingly, especially if you have not reached menopause.** The pre-menopausal breast is extremely sensitive to radiation, and each mammogram exposes the breast to significant amounts of radiation. Research has shown an increase in the incidence of deaths from breast cancer among women who had mammography before they reached menopause. In addition, other studies have suggested that the tight compression of the breast that occurs during mammogram may promote the spread of pre-existing cancer cells. ***Mammograms are not harmless!***

- **Learn proper breast self-examination.** Remember that 90 per cent of all breast cancers are discovered by women themselves who do self-examinations. A new device called the *Sensor Pad* increases the reliability rate of self-examination. Explore your options.

> **The health of your breasts is in your own hands.**
> **Start your breast cancer prevention program today!**

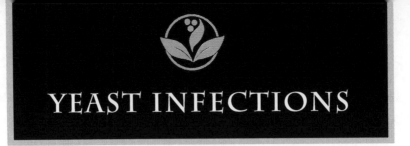

YEAST INFECTIONS

When you are told that you have a yeast infection this usually refers to an infection caused by a type of yeast called Candida albicans. The Candida organism is normally present, along with many other bugs and critters, in the digestive tract and the vagina of healthy women. Usually, they live together in peace and harmony and cause no problems.

In certain circumstances this delicate relationship is disturbed and the yeast can overgrow and infect the mucous membranes, commonly in the vagina and mouth. In some instances, Candida can even invade the blood and deeper tissues causing a wide variety of serious problems.

Woman (and men) may sometimes develop a Candida infection after taking antibiotics. The antibiotics kill the bacteria that normally keep the Candida under control, allowing the Candida organism to grow unchecked. Pregnant women, diabetics and obese people are particularly prone to Candida infections. Steroid medication, including certain skin creams, can also promote growth of Candida.

In some women, hot sweaty conditions or the use of tight underwear made from synthetic materials may trigger off yeast infections. In others, stress and emotional factors like a dysfunctional sexual relationship may be the underlying cause of recurrent vaginal yeast infections. Still others tend to have infections just before their menses, which suggests a hormonal imbalance.

COMMONLY AFFECTED AREAS

Vagina

The vagina is the most common site of Candida infections. Most women will have a few episodes of a vaginal yeast infection (vulvovaginitis) during their lifetime. This occurs most often, however, in women who are pregnant, those taking antibiotics or steroid medication, or those with diabetes. Typical symptoms include a thick, white or yellow vaginal discharge, with burning, itching and redness on the walls and the external areas of the vagina.

Skinfolds

This includes under the breasts, in the groin area, the navel and the anus. Symptoms include a rash with patchy areas that may ooze whitish fluid. The area will itch or burn. Candida infections may also occur at the corners of the mouth, creating cracks and tiny cuts. This is often caused by ill-fitting dentures.

Mouth

Thrush is a Candida infection of the mouth. Creamy white patches will appear on the tongue or sides of the mouth. Thrush can appear in a healthy child; however, in an adult it may be a symptom of a more serious disorder such as diabetes or AIDS. The use of antibiotics can also cause thrush.

Nail beds

Paronychia is caused by Candida growing in the nail beds of the fingers and toes resulting in a painful swelling and secretion of pus. Infected nails become disfigured, may turn white or yellow and may separate from the surrounding skin. Diabetics and women who constantly have their hands in water are particularly prone to this problem.

Penis

Uncircumcised men who have diabetes or whose sexual partner has a vaginal Candida infection are at risk. A red, itchy, scaly, often painful rash appears on the head or the underside of the penis. However, it is important to note that an infection of the penis (or vagina) may not always cause obvious symptoms and partners may unknowingly continue to reinfect each other.

CONVENTIONAL TREATMENT

Treatment depends upon the location of the yeast infection. Infection of the skin is treated with medicated creams and lotions containing anti-fungal drugs, for example, Nystatin. Nystatin works only on the skin and membranes and in the bowel and is not absorbed into the system. Suppositories may be used for vaginal and anal infections. Medication for thrush may be taken as a liquid swished around the mouth or as a slowly dissolving lozenge.

In severe cases, powerful systemic anti-fungal drugs in tablet form may be prescribed, for example, Diflucan. This form of treatment should be carefully monitored by your doctor, as serious side effects can occur from long-term use.

Conventional physicians often encounter the particularly vexing problem of women who have multiple vaginal yeast infections that are difficult to control. Many of these women are treated with multiple courses of potent anti-fungal drugs, often without relief. This situation often responds to a more natural approach.

THE NATURAL APPROACH

Correct predisposing factors

These are mentioned above – diabetes, hormone imbalance or stress. Careful attention to personal hygiene and the involvement and treatment of your sexual partner is important.

Correct your diet

This is critically important. If you have a chronic yeast problem, failure to change your diet will result in failure to resolve the issue. Anyone who tells you that you can just take an anti-fungal drug to cure the problem is sadly mistaken!

Removal of sugar, including honey and sweet fruits and their juices, from the diet cannot be overemphasised. Candida thrives on sugar. Many patients suffering from this problem have serious sugar and carbohydrate cravings that are of an addictive nature. There is no magic bullet. Dairy products and yeast-containing products (that includes all baked goods – breads, biscuits and so on) are also a definite no-no.

I suggest that you eliminate these foods entirely during the recovery period and possibly reintroduce them slowly after you have been free of infections for at least three months. If you have food allergies, those foods need to be avoided also. The book, *The Yeast Connection* by Dr Crook offers a specific anti-Candida diet. I recommend supplementing your diet with the Cellular Nutrition Program.

Support your immune system

Strengthening the immune system is crucial. The natural antioxidants, vitamins A, C and E and the mineral selenium (the ACES), along with herbs like schizandra and rosemary are excellent immune system boosters. Adequate rest and good stress management are equally important.

Take natural anti-fungal agents

- **Probiotics**

Taking certain healthy bacteria is beneficial in the prevention and treatment of yeast infections of the intestines and vagina. These bacteria normally live in the intestines and vagina and keep the unhealthy germs under control. They are called probiotics (in contrast to antibiotics) and are particularly useful in treating the yeast syndrome. The most popular of these are the Acidophilus and Lactobacillus bacteria. I use a product called Flora Fiber in which the bacteria are combined with fibre. This is a healthy way to restore the natural balance to the body without the use of powerful drugs.

- **Herbs**

Garlic has a direct yeast-killing effect and should be used liberally in cooking. Goldenseal (as a tea) and oregano (as an oil) are herbs that also have anti-fungal properties. Aloe vera provides tremendous healing benefits to the intestinal tract. As part of the treatment of a yeast infection it should be taken two or three times daily before meals.

Detoxify the system

A program of cleansing, including colon hydrotherapy, done regularly every three months, is useful in preventing a recurrence of yeast infections.

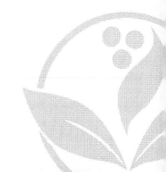

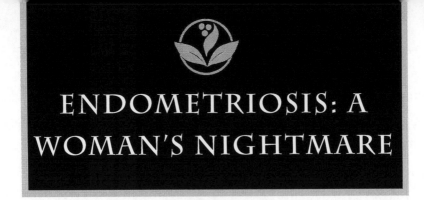

ENDOMETRIOSIS: A WOMAN'S NIGHTMARE

More and more women are being diagnosed as having a mysterious disease called endometriosis. Dr John Lee, an expert in the condition, described endometriosis as being a serious female condition in which tiny clusters of endometrium (cells lining the inside of the uterus) become scattered in areas where they don't belong – the ovaries and fallopian tubes, within the wall of the uterus itself (adenomyosis), on the outer surface of the uterus and other pelvic organs, the colon, the bladder, the sides of the pelvic cavity, and even to distant sites like the lungs or the umbilicus.

With each monthly cycle, these islets of endometrium respond to hormones exactly as endometrial cells do within the uterus: they increase in size, swell with blood, and bleed into the surrounding tissue at menstruation. This bleeding (no matter how small) causes inflammation and is very painful, often disabling.

Symptoms begin seven to twelve days before menstruation and then become excruciatingly painful during menstruation. The pain may be diffuse and may cause painful intercourse or painful bowel movements, depending on the areas involved. Women with endometriosis are often unable to conceive. Diagnosis is not easily established, as there is no blood test to identify abnormal endometrial tissues. Laparoscopy (a surgical procedure that enables a doctor to look into the abdomen with a small scope) is often resorted to for diagnosing this problem.

WHAT CAUSES ENDOMETRIOSIS?

While gynaecologists are still debating the cause, what is certain is that the hormone oestrogen stimulates endometrial tissues. I consider endometriosis to be another disorder of **oestrogen dominance**, that is, too much oestrogen and/or too little progesterone. It is caused by the same hormonal imbalance that can result in uterine fibroids, breast lumps, breast cancer, PMS, ovarian cysts and many of the symptoms of menopause. This is why during pregnancy endometriosis recedes, only to recur after the pregnancy when normal periods return. The higher levels of progesterone during pregnancy temporarily correct the oestrogen dominance.

CHEMICAL OESTROGENS

Endometriosis seems to be a disease of the twentieth century. Chemical oestrogens known as xenoestrogens (xeno means foreign) first came to widespread scientific attention in the early 1990s. Researchers found a link between exposure to chemicals with oestrogen-mimicking effects (even at very low concentrations) and endometriosis. These oestrogen mimicking chemicals may be found in everyday materials such as the varnish coating the inside of food cans, laundry detergent and plastic water bottles.

Research at the University of Wisconsin on monkeys in 1993 showed a strong link between exposure to the chemical dioxin and endometriosis. Dioxin is a by-product of pesticide production and use, and of pulp and paper manufacturing. This chemical can also be produced through the burning of hazardous waste. It can lead to oestrogen dominance that increases a woman's risk of developing endometriosis. The greater the exposure to dioxin, the more severe the endometriosis risk. German scientists had also confirmed an association between PCB (another xenoestrogen) contamination and endometriosis.

CONVENTIONAL TREATMENT FOR ENDOMETRIOSIS

Mainstream treatment of endometriosis is difficult and not very successful. Surgical removal of each and every endometrial islet throughout the body is often unsuccessful. Many of the tiny masses are simply too small to see, and eventually they enlarge and the condition recurs.

More radical surgery – the removal of both ovaries, the uterus and the fallopian tubes – is not a pleasant prospect. Other medical treatments attempt to create a state of pseudo pregnancy, using drugs called progestins to simulate the high progesterone levels of pregnancy.

THE ALTERNATIVE APPROACH

This approach deals with the underlying basis of the problem rather than just managing the symptoms.

- Detoxify the body to remove oestrogen-like toxins that may already be present. There are a number of detoxification techniques available.

- Eat a primarily plant-based diet to avoid the hormone-like chemicals in commercial meat, poultry and dairy. Limit the consumption of refined and concentrated carbohydrates (such as sugar, white flour, fruit juices and dried fruit). Alcohol, caffeine, and chocolate should also be avoided. There has been convincing research on food and beverages with a high sugar content, and their relation to menstrual cramping and associated pain. The cruciferous vegetables and soy are particularly helpful in oestrogen balancing.

- Take nutritional supplements. The Cellular Nutrition Program is very useful. Specific agents like the omega-3 fats, vitamins E, C and the Bs, magnesium and zinc and the herb Tang Kuei all help relieve inflammation and pain.

- Employ healthy stress management techniques. Chronic stress adversely affects the delicate hormone balance and worsens the problem.

- Use a natural progesterone cream. Bio-identical progesterone as a skin cream (not a progestin drug) can be safely administered to create levels similar to those of pregnancy. This cream is administered from day 8 to day 26 of a normal 28-day menstrual cycle. This treatment is often effective in relieving the symptoms of endometriosis. The goal is to find the lowest dose of natural progesterone cream necessary to control your symptoms. It is very important to choose a cream of high quality and potency.

This treatment requires patience and the direction of an experienced wellness practitioner. Over time (four to six months), however, the monthly pains gradually subside as monthly bleeding in the islets becomes less and healing of the inflammatory sites occurs. The monthly discomfort may not disappear entirely in all cases but will at least become far less. Endometriosis is ultimately cured by menopause but could be prevented by lifestyle choices.

This alternative technique is surely worth a trial, since the conventional alternatives are not all that successful and are laden with undesirable consequences and side effects.

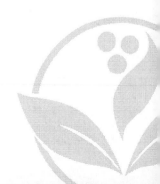

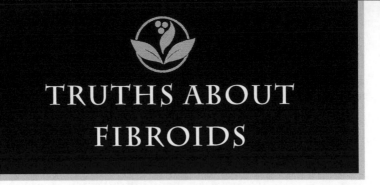

TRUTHS ABOUT
FIBROIDS

WHAT ARE FIBROIDS?

Fibroid, uterine fibroid, tumour, fibroid tumour, growth, fibroma, fibromyoma, leiomyoma. All of these are different names for a condition that may affect as many as 80 per cent of Jamaican women. In Jamaica and most western countries the most common surgery performed on women is the hysterectomy (removal of the uterus). In the United States 600,000 women lose their wombs each year to the gynaecologist's scalpel. In Jamaica (and elsewhere), the commonest reason for this female surgical castration is uterine fibroids.

Fibroids are non-cancerous tumours of the uterus that grow out of the muscle cells that form the walls of the womb. They can be as small as a pea or as large as a watermelon.

Amazingly, very little research is being done on the cause of fibroids. All the attention (and money) is directed at treating the condition after symptoms developed. This is a poor reflection on modern medicine.

FIBROID FACTS

Here are some facts, along with my own observations, about fibroids.

- Four out of five women have fibroids but only about 25 per cent of women have fibroids that cause troublesome symptoms. Many fibroids remain small and cause no trouble. However, it is easier to get rid of the problem when the fibroids are small. The usual advice given to women with small fibroids to 'just watch them' is, to my mind, ridiculous. Problems usually arise between ages 30 and 50, but younger and younger Jamaican women are now being afflicted. We need to tackle the problem as early as possible.

- Black women who adopt a western diet and lifestyle are twice as likely as Caucasian or Asian women to have fibroids.

- Each fibroid is derived from a single cell in the womb that begins to multiply abnormally. The cell begins misbehaving because of abnormalities that develop in its chromosomes. Hormone imbalance influences the behaviour of chromosomes.

- Changes in a woman's hormonal balance influence the development of fibroids. The hormones oestrogen, progesterone and probably insulin are mainly involved.

- Fibroids grow rapidly during pregnancy when hormone levels are high and shrink after menopause when hormone levels are low.

- All the hormone-sensitive organs in the body – the uterus and breasts (and prostate in men) – are now plagued by fibroid-like growths.

- Modern women (and men) are now being exposed to unnatural hormones (mostly oestrogen-like) in unprecedented ways. Many animal foods are laced with hormones while many pesticides, industrial chemicals, drugs, dyes and even some personal care items, like shampoos, contain hormones.

- A high consumption of commercial, non-organic meats is associated with an increased risk of fibroids.

- A plant-based diet, high in soy and organic green leafy and cruciferous vegetables, is associated with a low incidence of fibroids.

- There is a relationship between obesity and fibroids. The fatter a woman is, the more oestrogen her body produces. Oestrogen fuels the growth of fibroids. Of course, not all women who develop fibroids are obese.

- I suspect that some of the dietary factors that cause blood sugar problems and diabetes also contribute to fibroids. Insulin is a growth-promoting hormone and many diabetics have high levels of insulin.

CONVENTIONAL TREATMENT

Many women are very reluctant to have their wombs cut out, while there are others that are extremely satisfied with this final solution. Each case is unique and I strongly recommend that, before making a decision for or against surgery, you have a frank and unhurried discussion with your gynaecologist. You should prepare for this meeting by writing down beforehand all the questions and concerns that you have. Ask about the more recent procedures, like uterine artery embolisation (UAE) and myolysis. Make sure you understand the difference between myomectomy (removal of the fibroids only) and hysterectomy (removal of the entire uterus).

CONSIDER THE ALTERNATIVES

These non-conventional therapies that I will now discuss have the following goals:

- To correct the hormonal imbalance that caused the fibroids
- To relieve the symptoms that the growth produces, that is excessive bleeding, pain or pressure
- To prevent further enlargement of the fibroid
- To encourage the shrinking of the fibroids in the longer term.

I am not acquainted with any alternative therapies that can make you pass out or expel your fibroid. Neither do I know of any that will dissolve or melt fibroids.

Diet

Switch to a plant-based diet, high in soy and organic green leafy and cruciferous vegetables like broccoli, cauliflower and cabbage. Minimise your intake of animal foods especially commercial red meats, dairy and poultry. Fish and soy should be the preferred source of protein. Avoid the simple and processed sugars and carbohydrates such as flour products, candy, pastries and soft drinks. Supplementing with vitamins, minerals and micronutrients is essential.

Correct obesity. The fatter a woman is, the more oestrogen her body tends to produce and oestrogen fuels the growth of fibroids. The Cellular Nutrition Program is an excellent way to meet the dietary requirements listed above.

Detoxification

Cleanse the body as much as possible of the pollutants and toxins that it accumulates from the food we eat, the air we breathe and the water we drink.

An effective cleansing program can include fasting, colon cleansing, sauna treatments, herbal cleansers and chelation therapy. Intensive detoxification should be done under the supervision of a trained health care provider.

Herbs

A number of herbs have been used effectively in controlling the problems associated with fibroids. These include Tang Kuei, chaste tree, ginger and black cohosh. Professional advice regarding dosage and administration is recommended.

Natural progesterone cream

Natural progesterone cream is a powerful way to balance the stimulating effects of excess oestrogen on the uterus. It contains the identical substance that your body produces in a cream that is applied to the skin. This is different from synthetic drugs (progestins) that try to copy progesterone, but have many side effects. Get some professional advice on using natural progesterone cream as part of your anti-fibroid program as it can greatly improve your results.

Castor oil packs

A particularly novel approach involves the use of castor oil packs for fibroids. Castor oil packs have been used for thousands of years throughout the world for a variety of ailments. My research has shown that castor oil packs can play a part in shrinking fibroids and relieving pain and discomfort. (See the chapter on Castor Oil Packs)

Stress management

Poor stress management worsens the symptoms of fibroids, as chronic stress will contribute to hormonal imbalance. An important part of your program involves finding time for rest and practising effective relaxation strategies. Many women are worried about cancer developing in the fibroids. I have never seen this happen. Please talk with your doctor for reassurance.

Finally, I suggest that you keep a notebook to record your symptoms and your own evaluation of how you are responding to the natural approaches recommended. This will help you discover what works best for you. Good luck with this common and sometimes distressing problem.

Modern western medicine deals with menopause as if it were a disease rather than a normal part of a woman's life. However, in many other cultures it is considered a natural and positive part of the life process. In societies with this philosophy, women do not experience the symptoms usually associated with menopause. For instance, detailed investigations of rural Mayan Indian women in South America revealed that they do not experience any symptoms of menopause, including osteoporosis. Mayan women view menopause as an event that not only makes them accepted as respectable elders, but also relieves them of the responsibility of having children. The researchers concluded that the main reason these women did not experience any of the symptoms associated with menopause, probably had to do with their attitude, that is, how they regard menopause.

Jamaican women, on the other hand, often refer to menopause as the 'change of life', and see it as a period of adjustment. Even though physiological factors are involved, menopause is more than a biological event, as social and cultural factors contribute significantly to how women react to it.

WHAT IS MENOPAUSE?

Menopause denotes a cessation of menstruation or 'periods' and usually occurs within a few years of the fiftieth birthday for most women. Twelve months without a period is the commonly accepted rule for diagnosing menopause.

SYMPTOMS

The common symptoms of menopause include:
- Hot flashes (excessive heat and sweating)

- Vaginal dryness
- Forgetfulness and poor concentration
- Frequent urinary tract infections
- Headaches
- Cold hands and feet
- Irritability, mood swings and poor sleep

CAUSE OF MENOPAUSE

Menopause is believed to occur when all the eggs in a woman have been depleted. At birth, a woman has about one million eggs in her ovaries. By puberty, the number decreases to about four hundred thousand. Only about four hundred of these eggs will mature during a woman's reproductive years. At the onset of menopause, the ovaries cease to function and this results in a reduction in the production of the main hormones – oestrogen and progesterone. Thus menstruation ceases. Interestingly though, other tissues, including the fat cells in the body, continue to produce some oestrogen. Surgery, drugs, radiation and some diseases may also bring on menopause.

NATURAL APPROACHES FOR MANAGING MENOPAUSE

The following methods can be used to manage menopause safely and naturally.

Get a routine medical check up

I recommend that at the start of menopause, you go in for a routine medical evaluation. This should include breast and pelvic examinations, blood tests of your hormone levels and, if indicated, a test for osteoporosis. This will provide a yardstick to measure changes in the future.

Pay attention to your diet

- Increase your intake of plant foods, especially those containing phytoestrogens (oestrogen-like substances in plants). This includes soy, nuts, whole grains, parsley and fennel. Eat lots of vegetables and fresh fruit.

Menopausal symptoms are rare in cultures where a predominantly plant-based diet is consumed.

- Decrease your intake of animal foods, dairy and hydrogenated vegetable oils.

Take supplements

Nutritional supplements, especially vitamins E and C, omega-3 fats and magnesium are helpful in reducing menopausal symptoms.

Take herbs

Many herbs help to balance the female glandular system. These include Tang Kuei, black cohosh, chaste berry, evening primrose and Ginkgo biloba. There is now scientific evidence to show how some of these herbs act. For example, black cohosh has been shown to balance a hormone called leutenising hormone, balance blood flow and reduce inflammation while Tang Kuei has been shown to improve the balance between oestrogen and progesterone in the body.

Lifestyle modification

There is an area in the brain called the hypothalamus, which controls many body functions including body temperature, metabolism, mood, stress reactions and hormones. Many of the symptoms of menopause seem to be related to alterations in the function of the hypothalamus.

Several natural lifestyle measures stimulate the body to produce substances called endorphins that balance the functions of the hypothalamus and can have a positive impact on the symptoms of menopause. These lifestyle practices include:

- Exercising: studies clearly show that regular exercise decreases the incidence of hot flashes and vaginal dryness associated with menopause.

- Not smoking: smoking significantly increases the risk of an early menopause while worsening its symptoms.

- Managing stress effectively: this makes this period of adjustment much easier.

Use hormone replacement therapy

This is a controversial issue, but, in my opinion, hormone replacement therapy (HRT) is very useful and safe if the following principles are followed:

- Have your hormones measured first to determine what needs balancing. A blood or saliva test of your oestrogen, progesterone, DHEA, testosterone and thyroid hormone levels should be done.

- Use bio-identical hormones. This means giving back to the body the exact substance that it normally produces rather than a drug that is not the same and that invariably carries a high risk of negative side effects. These identical hormones are best administered as a cream or gel that is absorbed through the skin. Oestrogen, progesterone and testosterone can all be given in this way and are available here in Jamaica. Natural progesterone cream is a particularly useful and safe alternative to the synthetic oestrogen or progestin drugs often prescribed.

- Monitor your hormone levels and adjust dosages to bring your levels to normal. Consulting a physician who is familiar with this approach will make this much easier.

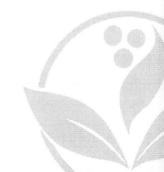

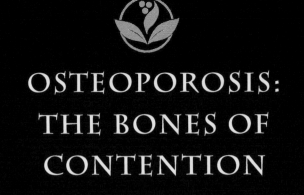

OSTEOPOROSIS: THE BONES OF CONTENTION

Osteoporosis is a condition characterised by a loss of bone mass and weakening of the bones. It has become big news and big business in today's world. Over the last 25 years or so, it has become a disease that is of major concern to women throughout the industrialised world. Advertising campaigns in the media and fact sheets in doctors' waiting rooms and pharmacies continually warn women of the dangers of disappearing bone mass.

The statistics from the United States say that over 20 million Americans (both men and women) have osteoporosis and approximately 1.3 million annually suffer a bone fracture as a result of osteoporosis. Sixteen per cent of patients who have hip fractures will die within six months while 50 per cent will require long-term nursing care.

Women are constantly bombarded with the message that the war on bone loss can be won with:

- calcium supplements and a daily consumption of calcium-rich foods, primarily dairy products.

- a doctor's prescription for long-term synthetic oestrogen for the post-menopausal woman, and, if additional help is required, add bone-building drugs like Fosamax.

Osteoporosis is a problem of bones, not women. Although men have half as many fractures as women they are more likely to die as a result of the fracture than are women. Yet little is said about men and osteoporosis. The 'male factor' was intentionally played down because it didn't fit with the definition of the condition as a woman's disease caused by lack of oestrogen. This strategy was necessary to promote synthetic hormone replacement. The truth is anyone can get osteoporosis.

THE BARE BONES ABOUT OSTEOPOROSIS

Bone is living tissue that undergoes constant transformation. Bone might appear to be static, but its basic components are continually renewed. At any given moment in each of us, there are between one and ten million sites where small segments of old bone are being dissolved and replaced by new bone. Bone tissue is nourished and detoxified by nutrients from the blood which is in constant exchange with the rest of the body. A healthy body will ensure healthy bones.

The conventional medical approach that focuses primarily on hormone replacement therapy, high calcium intake and prescription drugs is, in my opinion, flawed. Osteoporosis is not just an ageing disease or a deficiency in oestrogen or calcium, but a degenerative disease of Western culture. We have brought it upon ourselves through poor dietary habits and lifestyle factors, and exposure to pharmaceutical drugs.

The Bantu of Africa have the lowest rates of osteoporosis of any culture, yet they consume less than 500 mg of calcium daily. The Japanese average about 540 mg daily, but the post-menopausal fractures so common in the West are almost unheard of there, even though the Japanese have one of the longest lifespans of any population.

Studies of populations in China, Gambia, Ceylon, Surinam, Peru and other cultures all report similar findings of low calcium intake and low osteoporosis rates. Studies in people in North and Central America failed to find a link between calcium intake and bone loss. While it is agreed that adequate calcium is absolutely necessary for the development and maintenance of healthy bones, it is also obvious from these studies that high calcium intake is not necessary for healthy bones.

A HEALTHY LIFESTYLE FOR HEALTHY BONES

Like so many diseases, osteoporosis is better prevented than treated. Here are my recommendations:

Avoid bone destroyers

Minimise your consumption of potentially bone-damaging substances like excess animal protein, salt, saturated fat and sugar. Alcohol, caffeine and tobacco are harmful to your bones, as are the popular 'sodas' and 'colas'. Many prescription drugs like steroids weaken your bones.

Have good, balanced Cellular Nutrition

There are at least 18 key bone-building nutrients essential for optimum bone health. If one's diet is low in any of these nutrients, the bones will suffer. They include calcium, phosphorus, magnesium, manganese, zinc, copper, boron, silica, fluorine, vitamins A, C, D, B_6, B_{12}, K, folic acid, essential fatty acids and protein.

The body uses minerals only when they are in proper balance. For example, girls who consume diets high in meat, soft drinks and processed foods, which have high levels of phosphorus, have been found to have an alarming loss of bone mass. Balance is the key. I strongly recommend the Cellular Nutrition Program as a simple way to achieve that balance.

Exercise regularly

More and more studies are validating the extremely beneficial effects of a regular weight-bearing exercise program in increasing bone density in post-menopausal women, as well as men. A recent study found that, within a 22-month period, women who exercised three times a week increased their bone density by 5.2 per cent, while sedentary women actually lost over 1 per cent. Effective strength-training includes such exercise as walking uphill, bicycling in low gear, climbing steps and training with weights.

Balance hormones naturally

Yes, good hormonal balance does contribute to bone health. However, I do not believe that synthetic oestrogen and synthetic progestins are the answer. I suggest that women and men approaching midlife have their hormonal profile done by a lab test and that they use bio-identical hormones to bring their levels back to normal. Often, skin creams of natural progesterone and testosterone are most appropriate and effective and make oestrogens less often required. DHEA and Human Growth Hormone are sometimes needed.

Get enough sunshine

Vitamin D is essential to bone health. Your body makes vitamin D when your skin is exposed to sunlight. This naturally-made vitamin D is more effective than the vitamin D available in supplements. Without adequate vitamin D, all the calcium in the world will not get into the bones in proper quantities. People of colour need more sunshine than white-skinned people, and research shows that many black persons, especially women, living in tropical countries like Jamaica are vitamin D-deficient and lack enough exposure to sunshine. The situation is even worse for blacks living in temperate countries.

I recommend a half-hour sunbath on most days for the average individual.

 Live a healthy lifestyle and maintain healthy bones.

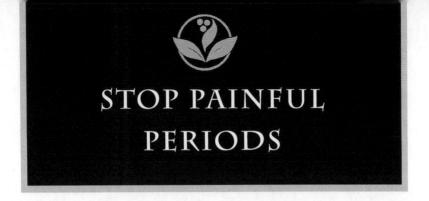

STOP PAINFUL PERIODS

Painful menstruation, referred to as dysmenorrhoea by doctors, is one of the most common health problems from which women suffer. As many as 90 per cent of women experience this problem. In over 10 per cent of women, the problem is so severe that they are unable to function normally while menstruating.

This condition translates into millions of dollars of lost wages and productivity as well as a significant decrease in women's quality of life for several days each month. One medical textbook estimated that painful periods cause the loss of over 140 million work hours each year in the United States. At the same time, billions of dollars are being made from the sale of pain killing drugs which do nothing to deal with the underlying cause.

In my view, dysmenorrhoea is, in most cases, a lifestyle related disorder having to do with nutritional, physical, hormonal and emotional imbalances. In a minority of cases, it may be the result of other medical conditions, like pelvic inflammation, fibroids and endometriosis, in which event those underlying problems should be treated. For the majority of sufferers, here is a natural 6-step plan.

6-STEP PLAN

Step 1: Nutritional program

Good nutrition at a cellular level gives your body the nutrients it needs to correct and heal imbalances and prevent cramps.

- A diet high in fresh vegetables and fruit, whole grains, beans, peas, nuts and fish is ideal.

- Drastically reduce or eliminate dairy products, meat, fried foods and other unhealthy fats, sugar, alcohol, added salt, MSG and other food additives.

- Start a program of nutritional supplements that includes soy protein, vitamins, minerals, trace elements and botanical factors. I recommend the Cellular Nutrition Program, as it provides all these elements in a simple combination.

Step 2: Special supplements

In addition to the general nutritional recommendations above, there are specific supplements that relieve cramps and prevent inflammation in a healthy, effective and natural way:

- The muscle relaxant herb Tang Kuei or angelica sinensis, has been used for thousands of years to prevent and relieve cramps. I use it in tablet form, which combines it with the calming, relaxing herb chamomile. It is most effective if taken throughout the month and the dosage increased just before and during the period. This combination is also a good general herbal tonic for females.

- Fish oil supplements that contain generous quantities of omega-3 fatty acids have natural anti-inflammatory and pain-relieving properties. Unfortunately, our diet tends to have an excess of omega-6 fats, which encourages the cramps and menstrual pains. Heavy dosages of fish oil capsules may be necessary to correct the imbalance.

- Calcium and magnesium supplements have powerful muscle relaxant and cramp-inhibiting properties.

- Mild diuretic herbs like celery, parsley, dandelion, sarsaparilla and uva ursi are useful in relieving the bloating, fluid retention and congestion some women experience.

- Ginger and ginkgo biloba will improve the circulation in the pelvic area and relieve nausea and vomiting.

- Individuals who have uterine fibroids will benefit from the use of castor oil packs. This novel therapy was covered in the chapter 'Truths About Fibroids'.

Step 3: Cleansing/detoxification

Cleansing the body, particularly the colon, is an important aspect of this 6-step program. Any congestion in the pelvic area will exaggerate menstrual pains. I recommend a high fibre diet along with fibre supplements, aloe vera and herbal cleansers. Colon irrigation therapy by a trained colon therapist can also be very effective.

Step 4: Relaxation and stress management

Painful periods are often a body/mind disorder. The condition is made worse by anxiety, fear, depression and stress. Your social conditioning and beliefs are also extremely important. Researchers have found that women who grew up in a household with women who had painful periods are much more likely to have painful periods themselves. Relaxation and stress management techniques and hypnosis can be extremely effective interventions. Aromatherapy that uses essential oils like lavender can relax you and relieve stress and tension.

Step 5: Exercise

Exercise promotes pain relief and prevents cramps because of its physical, psychological and hormonal benefits. I particularly wish to extol the benefits of yoga with its emphasis on deep breathing, tension relief, muscle relaxation and body awareness.

Step 6: Hormone balancing

An imbalance between the main female hormones – oestrogen and progesterone – can cause painful periods and severe bouts of premenstrual syndrome. The administration of natural hormone supplementation with natural progesterone cream, under a doctor's supervision, can be very helpful along with the herb Tang Kuei.

Instead of just popping pain tablets each month, consider starting this 6-step program and help your body balance and heal itself.

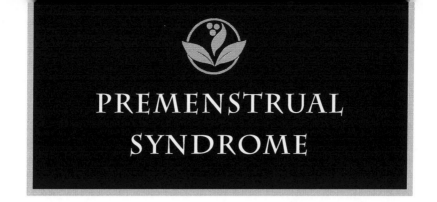

PREMENSTRUAL SYNDROME

*'One day she is all smiles and gladness, but the next she is
dangerous to look at or approach.'*
– Simonides, Greek poet, 400BC

The term PMS or premenstrual syndrome refers to both the physical and mental symptoms which occur before a woman's menstruation. Recently, the term premenstrual tension (PMT) has been used in reference to just the emotional changes. Up to one third of women have some symptoms, but in up to 5 per cent the problem is severe or incapacitating.

SYMPTOMS OF PMS

By definition, PMS symptoms occur in the two weeks each month before menstruation. Some women have PMS from the time they begin having periods but for most, PMS begins in the pre-menopausal years, around the mid-thirties, and becomes increasingly severe as the years go on. Although it's possible to list dozens of PMS symptoms, the most common are bloating/water retention and the resulting weight gain, breast tenderness and lumpiness, headaches, cramps, fatigue, irritability, mood swings, anxiety and a craving for sweet or salty foods. In women with severe PMS, irritability and mood swings can become outbursts of anger and rage. Existing conditions such as depression, asthma, allergies, and epilepsy can also become worse premenstrually.

Period pain itself is not included as a symptom of PMS. PMS lumps together a vast collection of symptoms and represents a mixed bag of individual responses to a natural event: the menstrual cycle.

CAUSES OF PMS

Many factors contribute to PMS. Stress, negative social attitudes towards menstruation, nutrition and lifestyle all influence hormonal changes and other bodily processes.

Along with many complementary medicine doctors, I believe that a hormonal imbalance called oestrogen dominance is the primary cause of PMS. It is one of the major factors causing not only PMS but also a long list of common female disorders like menopausal symptoms, uterine fibroids, breast lumps and endometriosis.

Oestrogen dominance

Oestrogen is one of the main female hormones which is produced in the ovaries. The other oestrogens are phytoestrogens, compounds in plants that have mild oestrogenic effects. Women who live in parts of the world where they customarily eat these plants will pass through menopause with hardly any symptoms whatsoever.

However, in modern times we now have very potent chemicals called xenoestrogens that we are exposed to on a daily basis. They can be found in the food we eat, the water we drink, the air we breathe and in the personal care products we put on our skin and hair. These are petrochemicals that act like oestrogen. They are extremely potent, even in very tiny amounts.

The other major female hormone is progesterone which balances the actions of oestrogen. In the latter half of each menstrual cycle, there is normally much more progesterone than oestrogen. So, if progesterone is low or missing, the woman will have a whole month of mostly oestrogen and will be described as being oestrogen dominant.

Women with PMS symptoms have low levels of progesterone. Their ovaries should be making progesterone, but they are not. These women are oestrogen dominant. The stress hormone cortisol makes oestrogen dominance even worse.

TREATMENT OF PMS

Correct oestrogen dominance

Avoid foods and drinks that contain oestrogens, such as commercial meats and poultry, household chemicals and personal care items with xenoestrogens. A diet high in fresh vegetables and fruit, high quality soy products and green tea helps in hormone balancing and is important. Use organic produce if possible.

Detoxify your body to remove existing offending chemicals. Far infra red saunas, colon cleansing and detoxifying herbs are very useful.

Use natural progesterone cream

Use natural progesterone cream under the direction of an experienced health care provider. This is the exact substance that is deficient in your body and not a chemical imitation. The popularly prescribed progestin drugs are not the same as the bio-identical progesterone in this cream and do not give the same results. The quality, the dosage and the timing of application of the cream are important for the success of the treatment.

Manage stress

This is critical, as poor stress management will result in high levels of the stress hormone cortisol that worsens oestrogen dominance. Stress commonly disturbs thyroid function and this should be looked out for.

Exercise, adequate rest, relaxation techniques, massage, reflexology, reiki, emotional release therapy and hypnosis are all useful tools.

Identify and avoid triggers

Activities or habits that trigger your symptoms are called PMS triggers. Examples include cigarette smoking, coffee, overwork, sugar, salty foods and some drugs. Keeping a diary of your symptoms can help you to identify these triggers.

Take supplements

The Chinese herb Tang Kuei helps relieve the symptoms of PMS as well as a variety of other hormone-related female disorders. Vitamins C and E, the minerals calcium and magnesium, the omega-3 fatty acids, the B vitamins, chamomile and St John's Wort are all recommended.

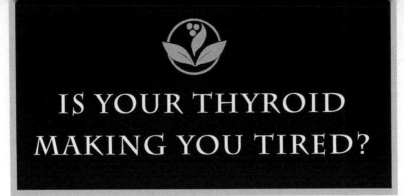

IS YOUR THYROID MAKING YOU TIRED?

Excessive tiredness or fatigue is the commonest complaint that patients today make to their doctors. Hypothyroidism, an underactive thyroid function, is a very common though often unrecognised cause of low energy levels. It is estimated that in the United States alone there are over 13 million people with undiagnosed low thyroid function.

The thyroid gland is a butterfly-shaped organ situated at the front of the neck, on both sides of the voice box or larynx. It produces thyroid hormones that serve many important functions including the control of body temperature, metabolism and energy production.

The common symptoms of low thyroid function include: low energy, weight gain, dry skin, constipation, hair loss, brittle nails, depression, irritability and intolerance to cold. Untreated, hypothyroidism can lead to serious health problems like heart disease, high blood cholesterol, osteoporosis, infertility, anaemia and recurrent infections.

ARE YOU AT RISK?

Women are seven times more likely to have this problem than men and although it can occur at any age, there are some times when women are especially at risk.

1. Just after having a baby, when depression, tiredness and failure to lose the baby fat are common symptoms

2. During menopause when a lot of symptoms blamed on low oestrogen levels may well be due to low thyroid hormone levels

3. After the age of 65, when symptoms of hypothyroidism like fatigue, memory loss and osteoporosis may be blamed on the ageing process.

Anyone having the above symptoms should have an assessment of their thyroid function done. Conventional medicine tends to depend on the results of blood tests to diagnose low thyroid activity although experts agree that blood tests alone are often misleading. The doctor needs to do a careful evaluation including a detailed questioning and examination of the patient. If this is not done, many cases will go undiagnosed. The blood tests may then assist in confirming the doctor's suspicion, but by themselves can be inconclusive.

A HOME TEST OF THYROID FUNCTION

You can have a good idea of the health of your thyroid gland by a simple at-home method of body temperature testing called the Barnes Test. Your body temperature reflects your metabolic rate, which in turn is largely influenced by thyroid hormones. Since activity increases your metabolism and therefore your body temperature, this test should be done while you're lying in bed, just after you have woken up. A simple mercury thermometer, available in pharmacies, is required for the test.

- Before going to bed at night, shake the thermometer down below 95° F, and leave it by your bedside.

- Upon awakening, place the thermometer in your armpit for a full 10 minutes (or two minutes for a digital thermometer). Remain still and reclined with eyes closed during the test.

- Read and record the temperature, date and time. Do this for at least three days.

- Menstruating women must perform the test on the second, third, and fourth days of menstruation. Men and postmenopausal women can perform the test at any time.

While a normal oral temperature is about 98.6° F, normal basal body temperature ranges between 97.6° F and 98.2° F. If your basal temperature measures consistently less than 97.8° F you may have a thyroid imbalance. Low basal body temperatures (that is, a positive Barnes Test), however, do not prove hypothyroidism by themselves. If your temperature is low and you have symptoms of an underactive thyroid, discuss the matter with your doctor to confirm the diagnosis and begin appropriate treatment.

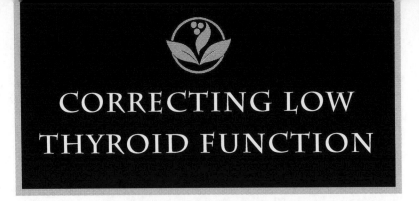

CORRECTING LOW THYROID FUNCTION

We have looked at how you may find out if your thyroid gland is underactive ('Is Your Thyroid Making You Tired?'). If it is, we should look for the underlying cause. In most cases of hypothyroidism, the thyroid gland is not producing enough thyroid hormone. What causes this?

CAUSES OF HYPOTHYROIDISM

Diet

The commonest cause used to be a deficiency of iodine in the diet that would often lead to an enlargement of the thyroid gland, called a goiter. With the widespread use of iodised table salt, iodine deficiency is now much less common. Goiters in people who have enough dietary iodine may be due to the excessive consumption of certain foods that block iodine utilisation.

These foods are known as goitrogens and include turnips, cabbage, mustard, cassava root, soybeans, peanuts, pine nuts and millet. Cooking usually renders these goitrogens inactive.

A wide variety of vitamins and minerals are also necessary for good thyroid function so good balanced nutrition is vital.

Immune system imbalance

Probably the most frequent cause of hypothyroidism today is a disturbance of the immune system. This condition is called Hashimoto's disease, named after the Japanese doctor who first described it. Here the body's own immune system attacks the thyroid gland and starts to destroy it. I strongly suspect that stressful situations (like pregnancy and menopause) as well as infections, environmental chemicals and certain food additives may contribute to this disorder. A special blood test can be done to diagnose the condition.

Doctors

Yes, a large number of persons are hypothyroid because of treatments given to them by their doctors for an overactive thyroid gland. These treatments include surgery, drugs or radiation. The subsequent damage to the gland that results is often irreversible. Looking for and dealing with the underlying cause of the hyperactive gland using natural methods can often prevent these severe treatments.

TREATMENT USING A HOLISTIC PROGRAM

- **A balanced diet.** This is essential. Ensure optimal intake of iodine, zinc, vitamins C, E and B complex. Ensure good levels of protein while minimising simple carbohydrates in the diet. Supplementing with the Cellular Nutrition Program is very useful. It contains additional nutrients like kelp, cayenne and Krebs cycle factors which improve the metabolism.

- **Immune system support.** Those with immune dysfunction, in particular, would benefit from supplementing with high dosages of antioxidants like vitamins A, C, E, selenium, the herbs schizandra, rosemary, pycnogenol, garlic and ginger. Large amounts of fish oil supplements will help heal any inflammation of the thyroid gland.

- **Stress management.** Low thyroid function is often triggered by stress, so learning to handle stress in a healthy way is most beneficial. Relaxation techniques should be used.

- **Exercise.** This increases the metabolism and has many other beneficial effects. Some yoga postures like the shoulder stand are particularly helpful as they stimulate, massage and increase the blood flow to the thyroid.

- **Medication.** This is the standard medical answer to hypothyroidism and a variety of synthetic drugs are used to give the body more of the lacking thyroid hormone. These are often necessary and very helpful. However, many holistic physicians, myself included, use natural thyroid hormone replacement instead. These are also prescription medicines but are made from desiccated animal thyroid glands. They contain a balance of all the thyroid hormones and often produce a better response. You may wish to discuss this option with your doctor. Changes in your basal body temperature readings (the Barnes Test described in the previous chapter) can be used as a guide in finding the appropriate dosage for you.

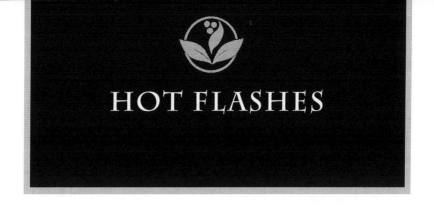

HOT FLASHES

The "hot flash" (HF), (also called a hot flush) is a very common complaint of women in mid life. It is experienced by up to seventy-five per cent of pre-menopausal and menopausal women in developed western societies. For some women the problem is minor, but for others, the HF is an extremely unpleasant and embarrassing sensation that can disturb sleep and interfere with daily life. By contrast, the problem is rare in many primitive societies where there is not even a word for the condition in some of their languages.

Although HF is mostly a female problem, men are also affected if the levels of the male sex hormone testosterone drop suddenly. Seventy-five per cent of men with prostate cancer who have their testes removed by surgery (orchiectomy) or who take medication to decrease testosterone levels, experience HF.

Typically, a hot flash is a sudden warm sensation often accompanied by a breakout of sweating usually confined to the upper half of the body – chest, neck, face and head. This may develop into an intense feeling of heat with the face, head and neck becoming flushed.

WHAT CAUSES THE HOT FLASH

Hormone Imbalance

The exact physiologic cause for HF is uncertain but the event is probably triggered by increased heat (or blood flow) to the heat regulatory area of the brain. The brain, sensing this heat, releases chemicals that cause blood vessels in the skin to dilate in an effort to release heat.

It seems that the sex hormones estrogens and testosterone normally allow the body to better tolerate changes in body temperature. When the levels of these hormones fall, anything increasing body heat or blood flow to the brain may cause a HF. The menopause and the andropause (male menopause), with its accompanying hormonal changes is the commonest cause of HF in both men and women.

Foods and Drinks

Foods and beverages, physically hot or containing spices like hot pepper can cause a HF. In this case, the heat directly stimulates and dilates the brain blood vessels. Alcohol, excess caffeine, other food additives or just eating a very large meal can cause HF. We still do not know all the different foods and food additives that can trigger this reaction. Cooling foods like fresh fruit and vegetables on the other hand will help prevent them.

Drugs & Surgery

Anti-estrogen drugs (e.g. Tamoxifen) often prescribed for breast cancer and anti-androgen drugs (e.g. Andracur) commonly used to treat prostate cancer may cause HF. Many other prescription drugs such as high blood pressure medicines, anti-depressants or anti-anxiety medications can also cause HF. In fact, all prescription and over-the-counter drugs should be checked to see if the HF is a known side effect. The B vitamin, niacin, may also produce flushing and heat in some people.

Stress

A very common cause of HF is a stress reaction that causes the release of adrenaline into the blood stream. This in turn causes increased blood flow and thus increased heat. A hot flash may then ensue. The stressful trigger can even occur subconsciously during deep sleep, probably while dreaming. This may explain the common occurrence of the HF at night.

Hot Environment

Another common cause of a HF is simply that the body is too warm. In general the warmer your surroundings, the greater the likelihood of you developing a HF. Research shows that menopausal women can reduce by almost fifty per cent the number of night sweats by lowering the temperature in the bedroom by a few degrees.

TREATMENT

First of all, if HF are mild or occur less that once per day, you might ignore specific treatment and focus on prevention strategies. There are also a number of other medical conditions that may produce HF, so get an initial evaluation from your health care provider.

Prevention

Look out for and try to avoid your own individual triggers i.e., strong emotions, stressful circumstances, excess caffeine, alcohol, cigarette smoking, hot food and drink, or hot environments. Drink enough water, usually eight or more glasses per day. Wear cool clothing made of natural materials. Exercise daily – walk, swim, dance or bicycle for thirty or more minutes, preferably in the morning.

Manage stress. Practise relaxation techniques like deep, slow abdominal breathing for fifteen minutes in the morning and evening. This can reduce the number of HF by as much as fifty per cent.

Hormone Replacement Therapy (HRT)

In my opinion HRT can be safely and effectively used to relieve HF if two important principles are employed. First, a hormonal profile should be done with a blood or saliva test. This will tell which hormone is needed and help in determining the right dosage. Second, only bio-identical hormones should be used. Progesterone, estrogens or testosterone may be then prescribed preferably as a skin cream.

Supplements

Soy based foods, omega-3 fats, evening primrose oil, magnesium and vitamin E are helpful supplements.

Herbs

Tang Kuei /Dong Quai Root

This well-known herb has been used for thousands of years in Chinese Medicine and has long been considered the women's ginseng. Traditionally used for hot flashes and other menopausal problems it is also useful for menstrual disorders through its antispasmodic action. I use Dong Quai in combination with the relaxing herb chamomile for these problems. This blend is available in a single tablet.

Black Cohosh Root

Black Cohosh is a phytoestrogen (plant estrogen) and is effective in eighty per cent of cases in relieving the symptoms of menopause when used consistently. Some authorities claim that it improves symptoms like HF, vaginal dryness and headaches as effectively as estrogen replacement therapy.

Chaste Tree Berry / Vitex

Vitex does not contain hormones but it acts on the pituitary gland, which stimulates the increased production of estrogen and progesterone. Vitex increases these hormone levels to help regulate the menstrual cycle and reduce menopausal symptoms.

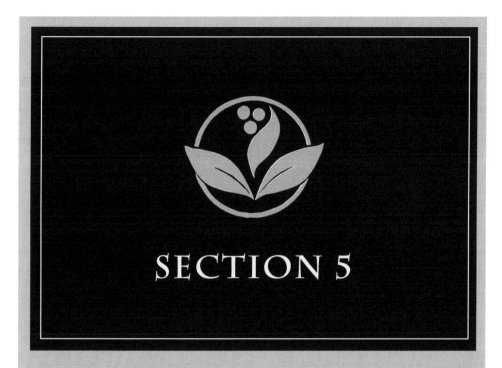

SECTION 5

DANGER
AREAS

'The best doctor gives the least medicines.'
– Benjamin Franklin

www.anounceofprevention.org

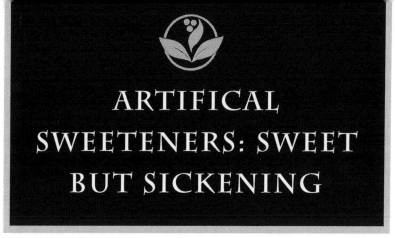

ARTIFICAL SWEETENERS: SWEET BUT SICKENING

The most popular artificial sweetener found in our supermarkets, kitchens, restaurants and on our very dining tables is aspartame. It is marketed under trade names like NutraSweet and Equal. In fact, you can hardly buy a stick of gum or a box of mints without being offered a dose of aspartame, and without reading the label like a hawk, you would not know because it's not always obvious that a product contains aspartame. On most restaurant tables right alongside the packets of white sugar, which is unhealthy in its own right, are pink and blue packets of artificial sweeteners which contain known poisons technically called excitotoxins.

Aspartame is a synthetic chemical composed of the amino acids phenylalanine and aspartic acid bonded with methyl alcohol. Methyl alcohol breaks down in the body to formic acid (the poison in an ants sting) and formaldehyde (embalming fluid). Each time you drink a diet soft drink or chew sugarless gum containing aspartame, you are feeding unhealthy doses of these substances into your system.

The amino acids can go directly to the brain and alter the function of your nervous system. Your brain naturally contains phenylalanine, but phenylalanine in high concentrations is very unhealthy. Aspartame consumption provides phenylalanine in excess to your brain. Researchers know that a rise in brain phenylalanine levels ultimately increases the risk of seizures. The other chemicals mentioned above are also very toxic. They are all excititoxins.

SOME ITEMS THAT OFTEN CONTAIN ASPARTAME

Aspartame is everywhere. Montesano, its main manufacturer has made a fortune from this chemical. Here is a list of common foods that often contain it:

Diet soft drinks, Instant breakfasts, Breath mints, Cereals, Sugar-free chewing gum, Cocoa and coffee beverages, Frozen desserts, Gelatin desserts, Juice beverages, Laxatives, Multi-vitamins, Milk drinks, Pharmaceuticals and supplements, No-sugar shake mixes, Tabletop sweeteners, Tea beverages, Instant teas and coffees, Topping mixes, Wine coolers, Yogurt, Children's vitamins.

ADVERSE REACTIONS AND SIDE EFFECTS OF ASPARTAME

As far back as the 1980s, the department of Health and Human Services in the US received over 10,000 complaints regarding adverse reactions to aspartame. One expert, Dr Janet Starr Hull, lists the following as some common side effects of aspartame use. These are tabulated here according to the parts of the body affected. (See table)

In spite of these adverse effects, the enormous power of vested economic interests contrived to 'prove' that aspartame was perfectly safe. Despite all the complaints, the FDA accepted the proof. Advertisements for aspartame portray it as a 'healthy' alternative to sugar. Such advertising makes aspartame even more dangerous to consumers who are ignorant of the artificial sweetener's potential side effects. Because of this deceptive advertising, people concerned about their health regularly use aspartame-sweetened products.

Instead of a healthy dietary and exercise program, people concerned with weight loss may use sugar-free foods sweetened with aspartame to reduce their caloric consumption. Unfortunately, aspartame is often associated with sugar cravings, overeating and weight gain!

MY RECOMMENDATIONS

- Develop the habit of carefully reading the ingredients list of everything you put in your mouth.

- Be particularly careful of 'sugar free' or 'sugarless' foods and beverages, especially diet soft drinks.

- The newest of the artificial sweeteners contains sucralose. I do not feel that we have enough experience with sucralose to be totally confident of its safety although, 'so far so good'.

Table: Effect of aspartame on various parts of the body

Part of the body affected	Effect
Nervous system	Epileptic seizures, Headaches, Migraines, Severe dizziness, Unsteadiness, Memory loss, Drowsiness and sleepiness, Numbness of the limbs, Slurring of speech, Hyperactivity, Restless legs, Facial pain, Tremors, Attention deficit disorder, Brain tumours
Eye	Blindness, blurred or decreased vision, Bright flashes, Decreased night vision, Pain in one or both eyes, Bulging eyes
Ear	Ringing or buzzing sounds, Hearing impairment
Brain	Depression, Irritability, Aggression, Anxiety, Personality changes, Insomnia, Phobias
Chest	Palpitations, Shortness of breath, High blood pressure
Intestines	Nausea, Diarrhoea, Abdominal pain
Skin	Itching, Hives
Respiratory system	Aggravated respiratory allergies such as asthma
Endocrine system	Poor control of diabetes, Menstrual changes, Thinning or loss of hair, Poor weight control, Low blood sugar, Severe PMS

- I recommend the herb stevia as a sweetener to my patients. Known in South America as the 'sweet herb', stevia has been used for over 400 years without ill effect. Stevia has been enormously popular in Japan, now rivalling NutraSweet, Equal and Sweet 'N Low. It is much sweeter than sugar, so a small portion of stevia goes a long way.

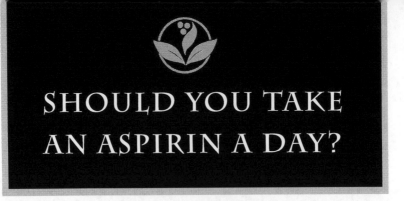

SHOULD YOU TAKE AN ASPIRIN A DAY?

WHAT IS ASPIRIN?

The common chemical name for this compound is acetylsalicylic acid (ASA). It was first synthesised in 1853 and the term aspirin became the popular generic name for the drug when it was trademarked by the German company, Bayer, in 1899. For the past 100 years, aspirin has been a preferred treatment for arthritis pain, headaches and fever. Today, many doctors recommend that the drug be taken on a daily basis for the prevention of heart attacks, the commonest killer today. It has been considered by some as the most successful drug in history.

ASPIRIN FOR HEART ATTACKS

The use of aspirin to prevent heart attacks is based on the drug's ability to inhibit the formation of blood clots or thrombosis in the body. Blood clots cause heart attacks by blocking the flow of blood through the coronary arteries into the heart muscle. The common saying 'aspirin thins the blood' is not strictly true; aspirin prevents clot formation by preventing blood elements called platelets from sticking together, a process that inhibits clot formation.

The widespread use of aspirin for the prevention of heart attacks is based on the results of several well publicised medical research studies. However, a number of respected scientists have questioned the conclusions drawn from those studies, but these views have not received equal publicity.

- Studies show that, although prophylactic aspirin may reduce the chance of a high risk individual getting a heart attack for the first time, there is no evidence that it will reduce the risk of a heart attack in low risk individuals or those without circulatory problems. In fact, the risks outweigh the benefits in the latter group. There is also no improvement in overall death rates in the people who take aspirin. There seems to be no justification for a relatively healthy individual taking aspirin 'just in case'.

- After a first heart attack, evidence shows that aspirin is useful for a period of time in preventing a second attack. The first aspirin tablet is normally taken as soon as possible after a heart attack. Then, in consultation with a doctor, a switch to low dosage enteric coated aspirin tablets (baby aspirin) is made. After four to eight weeks, if no further attacks threaten, I recommend that patients discuss stopping aspirin therapy with their doctors. This is because aspirin has serious side effects. Just look at this list: gastritis, peptic ulcer, intestinal bleeding, haemorrhagic shock and sudden death. Aspirin can also affect your eyes, increasing the risk of macular degeneration, a leading cause of blindness. There is even up to a 500 per cent increase in the risk of cataracts in individuals below age 55 who have been taking aspirin over the long term.

- These negative effects of aspirin were unlikely to have shown up in the studies because buffered aspirin was used. Buffered aspirin reduces the side effects of aspirin. It contains a significant amount of magnesium, a natural substance that contains its own powerful protective properties. Perhaps this is what is providing some of the benefits.

SAFER ALTERNATIVES

The most important protection against heart attacks is a healthy lifestyle. Excellent cellular nutrition, weight control, exercise, avoidance of cigarette smoke, stress management and adequate rest are all vital.

- Vitamin E at dosages as low as 100 to 250 IU daily has demonstrated impressive results in preventing a first heart attack, with side effects so minimal as not to be mentioned. Vitamin E at a higher dosage of 400 IU daily was also effective in protecting heart attack sufferers from a repeat attack.

- There is circumstantial evidence that **magnesium** is very important for heart attack prevention. Most heart attack victims at post mortem examination are found to be magnesium deficient. Although adequate studies on magnesium supplements for the primary prevention of heart attacks are not available, the experience of a number of clinicians and studies on the magnesium content of drinking water and heart disease make a good case for taking magnesium supplements. I recommend magnesium aspartate capsules, 200 to 400 mg daily.

The medical establishment has already accepted the use of magnesium in treating high blood pressure, heart attacks and heart failure.

Although this may seem a complex issue, I hope readers recognise that there are safe alternatives to aspirin that they can choose to protect and maintain a healthy heart. For the inevitable questions that will arise from my professional colleagues, I would refer them to an excellent review article published in the *Journal of Scientific Exploration* (Vol. 14, No. 4).

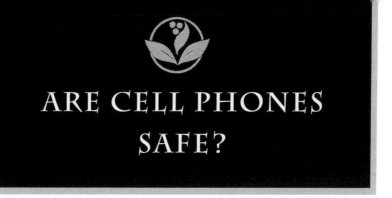

ARE CELL PHONES SAFE?

In the past few years, a technological and cultural revolution called the Wireless Age has exploded worldwide. There are now more than 1.5 billion cellular telephones in use around the globe, with Jamaica boasting more than its fair share. Here, everyone seems to use a cell phone. But, are cell phones safe or are they the cigarettes of the new millennium?

In the mid-20th century, doctors regularly advised patients to take up smoking to aid in weight control. The notion that inhaling tobacco smoke could be harmful was regarded as alarmist, unfounded, almost superstitious. A few generations later, smoking is now universally recognised as deadly, as it has been found to contribute to lung cancer, several other cancers and smoking-related heart disease, which are among the top causes of death. Today we shake our heads at our earlier stupidity.

Currently, millions of people are using cell phones – highly compact ultra-high-frequency transceivers with antennas that just happen to be situated directly above the ear when the device is in use. Like cigarettes in the last century, the safety of the long-term use of cell phones has not yet been demonstrated.

In May 2005, a legal precedent was set in the US. A California resident, Sharesa Price, whose job involved using a cell phone several hours each day, developed a brain tumour. She convinced the courts that her illness was caused by radio-frequency radiation from a cell phone, and was awarded US$30,000 for medical expenses.

Price now speaks to school assemblies and children about the need to use a headset when talking on a cell phone. She says, 'We need to explain to people that just like putting on condoms, you have to take this precautionary measure to make the product be as safe as it can be.' (*South Florida Sun-Sentinel*, October 2, 2005)

In 1993, Dr George Carlo, a public health scientist, was given US $25 million by the cell phone industry to do research that would reassure the public about the safety of their products. When his studies began revealing worrying trends, he was dismissed. His book, *Cell Phones – Invisible Hazards in the Wireless Age*, should be compulsory reading for our local health and technology leaders. Here are some of his findings:

1. Damage to the blood-brain barrier

The brain is extremely sensitive to chemicals. To survive and maintain brain function, humans have developed specific protections for the brain. One such protection is a special filter that keeps harmful chemicals from entering the brain. It is called the blood brain barrier. Radio-frequency radiation emitted from the antennae of mobile phones interferes with the blood brain barrier, and allows toxic substances access to the tissues of the brain.

2. Genetic damage

There is conclusive evidence from several researchers that the radiation from cell phones causes genetic damage to human blood cells. This damage leads to an increased risk of cancer.

3. Headaches

The more one uses a cell phone, the greater the occurrence of headaches, dizziness and general feelings of discomfort. Increasing the use of these instruments from less than two minutes to over 60 minutes per day, for example, made symptoms worse by over 600 per cent.

4. Cancer

Studies in the US, Canada and Poland of people exposed to radio-frequency radiation indicate an increased risk of brain, lung and blood cancers. The experts, however, agree that more specific research on cancer in cell phone users is urgently needed.

5. Motor vehicle accidents

There is a statistically significant increase in the risk of death due to motor vehicle accidents among users of mobile phones, regardless of whether the phone was handheld or had an external antenna.

6. Radiation in children

The radiation that emanates from a cell phone antenna penetrates much deeper into the heads of children than adults. Once it penetrates children's skulls, it enters their brain and eyes at an absorption rate far greater than it does in adults. These differences are profound and signify potentially serious health risks to children. Sadly, this did not prevent major players in the cell phone industry from mounting major advertisement campaigns targeting children.

RECOMMENDATIONS

Because cell phones are such an important part of modern life and modern communication, and so widely used, we need to find a way to coexist with them at minimal risk to our health. Here are some recommendations for doing so.

Restrict cell phone use and use a headset

- Add up the number of minutes you spend using a cell phone daily and try to cut down by 30 per cent or more.

- Keep the antenna away from your body by using a phone with an earpiece or headset. Everyone should routinely use a headset with his or her cell phone. I believe that everyone who buys a cell phone should be given a headset by the manufacturer free of cost.

- If you must use a phone without an earpiece, extend the antenna as much as possible. When the antenna is recessed inside the phone, the entire instrument functions as the antenna and the radiation is emitted from the entire phone into a wider area of your head, jaw and hand.

- Children under the age of ten should not use wireless devices of any type.

- When the signal strength is low, for example, inside some buildings, do not use your phone. The lower the signal strength, the greater the radiation emitted from the antenna.

- Do not use handheld phones while driving a vehicle.

Increase your body's resistance to radiation

- Eat lots of fresh vegetables and fruit. Use the Cellular Nutrition Program I use myself for optimal nutritional support.

- Supplement with the antioxidant ACES – vitamins A, C, E, and the mineral selenium.

- Supplement with schizandra, rosemary, ginkgo biloba, pycnogenol and garlic.

- Avoid cigarette smoke, alcohol, chemical pollutants, and other sources of radiation like microwave ovens.

- Get lots of fresh air, clean water and sunshine – natural healing tools.

- Do a detoxification/cleansing program every three to four months.

Remember, your health is in your hands, especially when you are holding a cell phone. The more powerful a tool, the greater its potential to help as well as harm.

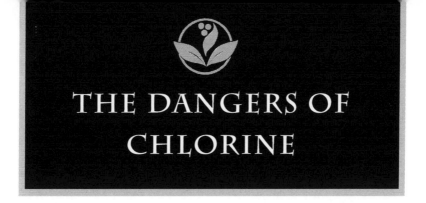

THE DANGERS OF CHLORINE

I am always recommending that you drink more water. But I suspect that, like most people, you don't enjoy the taste of chlorine in your drinking water. You only put up with it because it kills germs that are harmful to your health.

The benefits of using chlorine as a sanitising agent are obvious. The use of this chemical in the treatment of drinking water is responsible for the elimination of diseases like typhoid and cholera, especially in developed countries. However, this water treatment agent has a darker side. While we thought we were preventing epidemics of one disease, were we at the same time creating others?

WHY IS CHLORINE HARMFUL?

When water treatment facilities use chlorine to kill germs, this powerful chemical also reacts with organic materials in the water. When you drink chlorinated water, chemical reactions may also occur with the food in your stomach. These reactions, whether in the water or in the stomach, produce poisons called **trihalomethanes (THM)**. Simple examples of these are chloroform and bromoform. According to the Environmental Protection Agency, these chemicals are present in most public water supplies. Some scientific studies link them to an increased risk of cancer. The US Council of Environmental Quality reports that cancer risks among people using chlorinated water are up to 93 per cent higher than among those whose water contains no chlorine.

Other studies suggest that THMs may cause problems in the reproductive organs, the heart, lungs, kidneys, liver and nervous system.

Your skin absorbs chlorine

Most readers may assume that the drinking of chlorinated water is the main route of exposure to the nasty chemicals described above. Not so. Studies at the University of Pittsburgh found less chemical exposure from drinking chlorinated water than from showering or washing your clothes in it. The study found that, on average, absorption through the skin accounted for 64 per cent of water-borne contaminants entering the body. This research reveals that drinking may not be the sole, or even primary, route of exposure.

By penetration through the skin, the chemicals can adversely affect the skin and hair. Chlorine bonds chemically with proteins in the hair, skin and scalp so that:

- the hair can become rough and brittle and lose its colour
- the skin can become dry and itchy
- sensitive areas in the eyes, nose, throat and lungs can become aggravated.

Inhaling chlorine while showering

As bad as the above sounds, the major health threat caused by these chemicals is when they are inhaled as air pollutants.

Hot showers can release these dissolved toxins into the air. The lungs will readily absorb contaminants like chlorine, trichloroethylene, chloroform and benzene, which then pass from the lungs into the bloodstream.

PREVENTING CHLORINE POISONING

While chlorinating public water supplies is perhaps the most convenient way to address the problem of water contamination, it does present serious problems. Many developed countries have switched to ozone (a form of oxygen) to purify their water supply in a safer, healthier way. Ozone is made cheaply from the oxygen in the atmosphere. Should we not consider this in Jamaica?

Until that happens (don't hold your breath), I suggest the following:

- Drink, cook and, if possible, bathe with chlorine-free water. This may be done by using spring water, rain water or bottled water that is certified to be chlorine free.
- Boil water to remove most of the potentially harmful chemicals present.

In some instances, boiling may increase the concentration of some chemicals.

- Treat your water with your own purification or filtration system. A variety of these units are now available for home use. They vary in price and efficiency, so do your own research before investing.

- If you cannot avoid using chlorinated water, make sure that you are supplementing your diet with lots of antioxidant vitamins and minerals (the ACES – vitamins A, C, E and selenium).

- Advocate that our water supplies, swimming pools, hot tubs, and so on, be free from chlorine as the sanitising agent.

 Remember, you are not only what you eat; you are also what you drink.

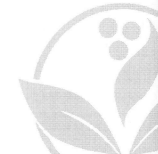

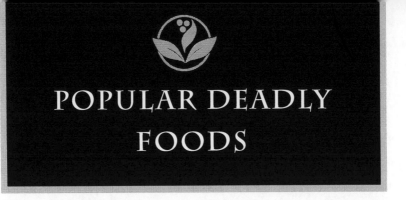

POPULAR DEADLY FOODS

Dr Joseph Mercola, a holistic doctor, believes that five very popular foods are unhealthy. I agree. Not only do some have very low nutritional value, but they may also give your body a dose of toxins. Here are five foods you need to be wary of.

SODAS

One can of soda has about ten teaspoons of sugar, 150 calories and 30 to 55 mg of caffeine. It is also loaded with artificial food colours, carbon dioxide and phosphoric acid. I can't think of any good reason to ever have it. The diet sodas that use harmful artificial sweeteners, like aspartame, create serious additional health problems.

Studies have linked drinking sodas to osteoporosis, obesity, tooth decay and heart disease, yet the average American adult drinks an estimated 56 gallons of soft drinks each year. We in Jamaica are not far behind. Drinking all that sugar water suppresses your appetite for healthy foods, and paves the way for nutritional deficiencies.

Soft drink consumption among children has almost doubled over the last decade, which is not surprising considering the millions of dollars spent by the manufacturers on advertising and marketing. If you routinely drink sodas, eliminating them from your diet is one of the simplest and most profound health improvements you can make.

DOUGHNUTS AND PASTRY

Doughnuts are fried, full of sugar and white flour and most varieties contain a particularly harmful type of fat called trans-fat. Commercial doughnuts contain as much as 40 per cent trans-fats. An average doughnut will give you about 200 to 300 empty calories, mostly from sugar, and very few other nutrients.

Many people have other pastries like a Danish as a snack at coffee breaks in the office. Nutritionally, this is one of the worst kinds of snacks. It is full of sugar, white flour and bad fats. It will cause blood sugar imbalances and will make you hungry again very soon.

FRENCH FRIES (AND NEARLY ALL COMMERCIAL FRIED FOODS)

Irish potatoes when consumed in excess are bad enough, as their starch is rapidly converted to glucose (blood sugar) that raises insulin in the blood and can devastate your health. But when potatoes are fried at high temperatures, all sorts of unhealthy things happen.

Anything that is fried, even vegetables, contains unhealthy trans-fats and a potent cancer-causing substance called acrylamide. Fried or barbequed meats will contain additional cancer-promoting substances like nitrosamines.

Foods that are deep-fried in vegetable oils, like canola, soybean, safflower and corn oil, are particularly problematic. These oils are very susceptible to damage from heat. Overheating a healthy oil can produce some unhealthy results.

It is theoretically possible to create a healthier French fry if you cook it in virgin olive oil or virgin coconut oil. Both these oils are healthy and extremely stable and are not damaged by the high temperatures of cooking.

CHIPS

Most commercial chips, corn chips, potato chips, banana chips, you name it, are high in trans-fats. Fortunately, some companies have responded to the warnings about trans-fats and have started to produce chips without trans-fats.

However, the high temperatures used to cook them will potentially cause the formation of carcinogenic substances like acrylamide, and this risk remains even if the trans-fats are removed.

FRIED NON-FISH SEAFOOD

Not all seafood is healthy. Deep-fried shrimp, clams, oysters, lobsters, and so on, have all the issues of the trans-fats and acrylamide mentioned above, plus an added risk of mercury.

These creatures feed on the bottom of the sea and are considered scavenger animals. They take in chemicals and germs that may be harmful. Seafood today is often contaminated with toxic mercury, and shellfish like shrimp and lobsters can also contain parasites and germs that may not be killed by cooking.

Eating these foods without due caution can give you four types of toxins – trans-fats, acrylamide, mercury and possibly parasites or bacteria. If you have a taste for seafood, have it steamed, baked or broiled and make sure shellfish is properly cleaned and cooked.

 Remember, you are what you eat.
Don't dig your grave with your teeth.

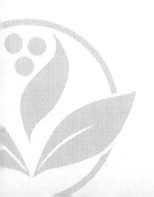

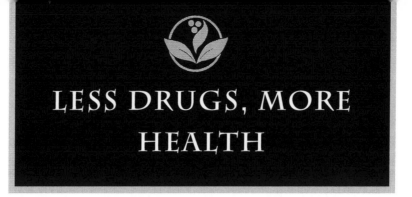

LESS DRUGS, MORE HEALTH

Today's society encourages a culture of heavy drug use. We warn our youngsters and athletes about the dangers of illegal drugs but turn a blind eye to the harsh reality that legally prescribed drugs kill and harm vast numbers of innocent victims every day. A recent report entitled 'Death by Doctoring' indicates that the number one cause of death in the US is now prescription medication (legal drugs). At the same time, Jamaican men, women and children are consuming more prescription medication than ever before. This is not a healthy sign. Though prescription drugs may sometimes save lives and alleviate suffering, they can also do great harm.

It was Benjamin Franklin who said, 'The best doctor gives the least medicines'. I would phrase that differently: 'The best patient needs the least medicines'. Anything that you can do to be healthier is likely to reduce the number and the dosage of drugs that your doctor would need to prescribe for you. A good doctor should certainly want the patient to take as little medicine as possible, as all drugs carry a risk.

MOST DISEASES ARE LIFESTYLE RELATED

Medical research clearly shows that most of our common diseases – heart disease, diabetes, high blood pressure, arthritis and many cancers – are the result of unhealthy lifestyles. They, in my experience, can often be prevented and even reversed by changing your lifestyle.

Simple non-drug interventions like optimal nutrition, vitamin, mineral and herbal supplements, exercise and effective stress management can, in most cases, restore health and prevent the progression of illness. Yet, it is not uncommon to find people taking as many as 15 different prescription medicines at the same time. Sadly, the majority of these drugs are meant only to manage the symptoms that the patients have but do not deal with the underlying cause of the problem.

DRUGS ARE DANGEROUS

The main reason that prescription drugs require a prescription is because they are potentially dangerous. Doctors try to carefully figure out just how much of the medicine you should take without causing undue danger. Despite this, 150,000 deaths occur each year in the US from patients taking drugs that their doctor prescribed for them!

Drug manufacturers provide information on drug safety for doctors. The patient can sometimes find this information in a leaflet included inside the box with their prescription. This information can also be obtained from a reference book called the *Physician's Desk Reference (PDR)*. The *PDR* is basically a 2,000+ page manual with details of every drug. It is easy to look up any drug that you or a family member may be taking. Be ready for some unpleasant reading. Most drugs have many more warnings and precautions than uses. In other words, drugs often have more dangers than benefits. In fact, some of the drugs commonly prescribed are needed to help counter the side effects of other medicines.

To make things worse, taking more than one drug at the same time can cause drug interactions – another set of dangerous problems due to the combination. The more you combine drugs, the more dangers you create.

DRUGS ARE BIG BUSINESS

Why then are so many drugs still used? Modern Western medical tradition is very drug oriented. There is a lack of emphasis on natural therapies in modern medical training. Most of the safe alternative treatments I use were not taught to me in medical school. I had to educate myself.

Money, big pharmaceutical industry money, is a huge reason. Look at the increasing number of pharmacies opening up all over the country. Selling drugs – legal or illegal – is big business. A second reason is that patients have come to accept and even demand drug therapy. They accept the risks and the side effects because they want a quick fix. If the doctor says it's okay then it is okay. 'Fix me up, Doc' puts the physician on the spot. The doctor has to do something, and since his/her background is in drugs and surgery, that is what he/she recommends. Of course, the public is continually being programmed by the massive advertising campaigns of the drug companies. This, in my opinion, is unethical and dangerous and some countries are considering banning this practice.

WHAT CAN THE PATIENT DO?

- Ask the doctor to fully explain the risks and side effects of any drug prescribed. Then ask for an explanation as to why you should take those risks. If you do not get a straight answer, or if the doctor is 'too busy' to discuss this with you, then it may be time to consider seeing another doctor.

- Ask to be given the lowest possible dose of the drugs prescribed. Get back to the doctor right away if there are any negative effects of the medication.

- Ask for possible non-drug alternatives! Some doctors are happy to work with interested patients who want to avoid medicines when they can. If your doctor is not interested, then you can find a doctor who is.

IF YOU ARE ALREADY TAKING MEDICATION

It is not a good idea to just suddenly stop medication. This is especially true if you are taking something more than a pain-reliever or other non-essential drugs.

- Share with your doctor that you are interested, if possible, in getting off the medicine that you are on or to decrease the amount that you have to take. It is best to work with the physician who prescribed the medicine for you in the first place. It is usually necessary for your doctor to monitor your progress while you carefully follow his/her instructions.

- If your doctor believes that you cannot reduce the level of your medication at all, you can honour that viewpoint without agreeing with it. A second medical opinion might then be in order. If several doctors all say 'Don't you dare stop taking your medication', then you need to do some serious reconsidering.

BOTTOM LINE

Drugs are common options for treating illnesses. They are, however, capable of doing significant harm, and great caution should be used in prescribing and taking these drugs especially for long periods. If proper nutrition and a healthy lifestyle bring you good health, then there may be no need for medication.

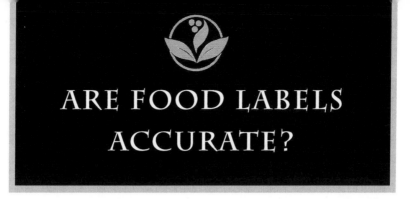

ARE FOOD LABELS ACCURATE?

Read food labels carefully. Educate yourself
about what you put in your mouth.

The modern food industry constantly invites you to eat more processed or packaged food. A major portion of your diet now comes out of a can, bottle, box, bag or package. Ideally you should be able to tell what is in the food you are eating by looking at the ingredients list and the nutrition facts label. However, this is not always the case and what you see on the label may not always be what you get.

FOOD LABEL INACCURACY

In the US and Jamaica most prepared foods sold are required by law to contain nutrition labels. In one US Food and Drug Administration (FDA) survey of nutritional labels, it was found that one out of every ten products had inaccuracies. They considered these results to be excellent.

A food label must be more than 20 per cent off in order for it to violate the law. This means that an item labelled as having 400 calories can legally have up to 480 calories. In addition, government food labs are allowed a 10 per cent margin of error in their tests.

Nutritional expert, Dr Joe Mercola, points out that some foods, particularly those making low-fat, low-carbohydrate or no-sugar claims, contain drastically different nutrients than are listed on the label. For instance, according to an ABC News report, two doughnut vendors that claimed their doughnuts were low-fat had dramatically understated the calorie and fat content of the doughnuts. In one case, a doughnut described as having 3 grams of fat and 135 calories was actually a chocolate doughnut that contained 18 grams of fat and 530 calories. Another product, chocolate chips, labelled as having zero carbs actually had 14.2 grams of carbohydrates.

HIDDEN AND MISLEADING INGREDIENTS

One of the most common misleading statements on food labels is 'No Cholesterol'. This statement can be found on many foods from vegetable oils to popcorn. When consumers read 'No Cholesterol' on a food label, most believe this brand is superior to another which does not make the claim. However, very few people know that cholesterol in your food plays a lesser role in affecting your blood cholesterol levels than the fat content of the food. Cholesterol and fat are not the same.

An even smaller number of people understand that only animal products contain cholesterol. All vegetable oils and margarines are cholesterol free, yet all are still 100 per cent fat. People mistakenly assume that low cholesterol means low fat. Certain French fries also claim to be cholesterol free. If the French fries were fried in a vegetable oil rather than lard this claim may be true. However, one French fry is still 15 calories, 40 per cent of which is fat.

Another misleading statement is the '100% vegetable oil' found on packages of crackers, cookies, margarines and shortening. Vegetable oils are mainly unsaturated fat which is 'heart healthier' than saturated fat. But if this vegetable oil is hydrogenated, the structure of the new fat is different and the body responds to it in a similar way as to saturated fat. Therefore, hydrogenated vegetable oil is not nutritionally better than saturated fat. It may be worse. Read the ingredients list carefully to see if the vegetable oil is hydrogenated.

Of course, the mother of all food label lies is found on your friendly carton of cow's milk. Milk labeled as '2%' really gets 34% of its calories from fat. The reason the dairy people lie and call it '2% fat' is that they sell more milk if people believe it is a low fat product rather than a high fat product. This is a blatant fraud on the consumer.

Be careful of products that proclaim 'No Salt Added' because it is not the same as 'Low Sodium'. No salt added refers to no table salt added. These products, therefore, may still contain monosodium glutamate (MSG) or one of the more than 60 other sodium-containing additives. Therefore, if you are on a low sodium diet, read the ingredient list to make sure it does not contain sodium in another form.

'Sugar Free' or 'Sugarless' does not mean the same thing as 'No Sugar Added' or 'Sweetened Without Sugar'. These are only a few examples of how the consumer can be misled.

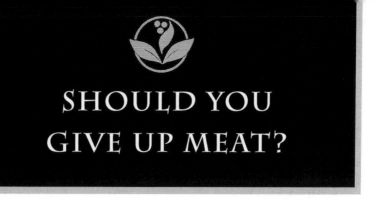

SHOULD YOU
GIVE UP MEAT?

Medical research published in the *Journal of the American Medical Association* has shown that heavy consumers of red meat have double the risk of developing colon cancer than those who consume smaller quantities of red meat.

But how does this compare to people who consume no red meat at all? Although the study does not say, I suspect that heavy consumers of red meat probably have at least four times greater risk of colon cancer compared to people who consume no red meat.

Research on total vegetarians (those who consume no animal products at all) suggests an almost total absence of colon cancer. When we consider that colon cancer is extremely common, accounting for 20 per cent of all cancers, these research findings become very important.

If medical research had suddenly announced the discovery of a new drug that would eliminate 20 per cent of all the cancers in the world, there would be no end to the publicity and fanfare it would be given in the media. Have you seen any headlines specifically promoting diet as the most effective anti-cancer strategy? No, that would not be in the best interest of powerful forces in the food and medical industries. But think of the lives that could be spared and the suffering and expense that could be avoided.

OTHER HEALTH RISKS OF RED MEAT

There are many health reasons to avoid eating red meat, and a higher risk of colon cancer is just one of them.

- The saturated animal fat found in red meat products contributes to heart disease and atherosclerosis.

- Commercial red meat contains contaminants such as heavy metals, pesticides, hormones and undesirable environmental pollutants that tend to collect in the fat tissues of the animal. These are absorbed into your body when you eat it. You can't eat red meat without getting some animal fat.

- Meat consumption may increase your risk of other cancers like prostate, breast and stomach cancer.

ENERGY/VIBRATIONAL RISKS

The energy/vibration of red meat concerns the environment in which the animal was raised. Was it a natural environment? Did the animal have access to open fields, sunlight and clean water? Or was it raised as part of a slaughterhouse operation, produced for the sole purpose of generating profits? If you eat meat that has undergone that kind of experience, you are consuming a product that is tainted with the negative experience of the animal from which it came.

ECONOMIC ISSUES

It takes ten acres of land to produce the same amount of red meat protein as it does for one acre of soybeans to produce an equivalent amount of plant protein. Producing a protein-rich plant called spirulina yields a tenfold increase over the production of soybeans. So think about it: one acre of farmland used to produce spirulina can produce 100 times as much protein as beef and red meat. That will be very important to realise as our world population grows and it becomes increasingly difficult to produce the protein required by the population.

SPIRITUAL/RELIGIOUS CONCERNS

Many religious traditions that promote non-violence and a deep reverence for life have spiritual motives for not eating meat. My own feeling is that individuals should be guided by their own consciousness (not the same as conscience) and not a prescribed dogma handed down from some authority.

There are indeed a lot of negative effects associated with the consumption of red meat, and this is why more and more people are now giving up red meat and moving to healthier foods like fish, free-range chicken or, better yet, plant-based proteins like soy foods – soy shakes, soy milk and tofu. This is where you'll get your best protective effect and disease prevention. You will also be helping to protect the environment at the same time, as less land is required to produce plant-based foods.

HOW TO TRANSITION FROM RED MEAT

Some people reading this are already following a plant-based diet, but others of you who might be considering making the change aren't sure exactly how to do it.

You want to start to reduce your consumption of red meat but not give it up completely yet, which is fine, since that's the way many people have done it.

- Decide how many times per week you will allow yourself to eat meat or declare certain days of the week vegetarian days.

- Decide on a period of time over which you will follow this dietary change, say three months, and then evaluate how you feel at the end of the period.

- It is also useful, though not essential, to do a cleansing of your digestive tract when you are changing your diet.

- Experiment with tasty and nutritious vegetarian foods.

These are just some ways to get rid of red meat in your diet, but there are many other ways and I encourage you to experiment and see how you'd like to approach it. The bottom line on red meat is that there is an increasing body of evidence supporting the notion that you may prevent cancer by pursuing a plant-based diet.

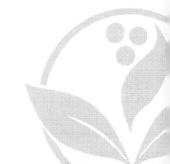

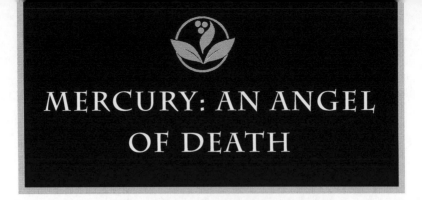

MERCURY: AN ANGEL OF DEATH

In Greek mythology, Mercury is the messenger of the gods. He ruled over wealth, good fortune, commerce and fertility. However, as a physical substance, mercury disrupts cellular function at all levels and robs the body of health and vitality.

Mercury belongs to a group of metals described as heavy metals. Mercury is a powerful poison that, even in small amounts, is more toxic than other heavy metals like lead, cadmium and even arsenic.

MERCURY POISONING

Exposure to mercury can cause damage to the nervous system, the brain, the kidneys, the liver and the immune system. Children and foetuses are particularly vulnerable. Some of the most common signs and symptoms of mercury exposure include irritability, fits of anger, lack of energy, low self-esteem, drowsiness, decline of intellect, poor self-control, nervousness, memory loss, depression, anxiety, shyness/timidity and insomnia. Recent research indicates that mercury also impairs heart and circulatory function.

Most poisons that enter the body are processed by the liver or kidneys and broken down into smaller components, then excreted in a less toxic form. Heavy metals are different. They cannot be broken down, so unless they are eliminated immediately, these absolutely indestructible elements accumulate and remain in the body as a source of potential damage.

Mercury is an unusual metal because it is a liquid rather than a solid, and it slowly evaporates at room temperature. Another name for elemental or metallic mercury is quicksilver. This is the kind of mercury used in thermometers.

Mercury, however, can combine with other chemicals to form organic mercury compounds such as those found in contaminated fish.

MERCURY IN YOUR MOUTH

The largest exposure to mercury among adults comes from a source that is completely avoidable – dental amalgam fillings that produce metallic mercury vapour. Metallic mercury in the fillings forms a gas that is highly volatile and readily inhaled. Every time you chew food or brush your teeth, mercury vapour escapes from these dental fillings into your mouth and lungs.

Today, there is no need for your dentist to put this poison in your mouth where it can so easily get to your brain. Ask for safer alternatives and consider having pre-existent mercury amalgam fillings removed. Sadly, the official line still taken by the dental profession is that mercury amalgam fillings are safe. I disagree.

MERCURY IN YOUR WORKPLACE

Mercury is still commonly used in dentistry, for the preparation of fillings; in laboratories and hospitals, as a reagent and fixative; and in medical instruments, electrical equipment, thermometers, barometers, pharmaceuticals, and some fluorescent light bulbs. It is also used in the manufacture of glassware and jewellery, and in the recovery of gold and silver.

MERCURY IN YOUR HOME

A report issued by the American Academy of Pediatrics addressed the hazards of mercury and suggested that pediatricians and parents should stop using mercury-containing thermometers. If the thermometer breaks, the mercury vaporises and can be inhaled, causing toxicity. The Academy calls for an end to the use of all mercury-containing thermometers. Also, because mercury has anti-fungal properties, it gets into homes as an ingredient added to indoor paints.

MERCURY IN BREAST MILK

Mercury can be passed from mother to child in breast milk. Studies have found a correlation between the mercury concentrations in the kidneys of newborn babies and the number of mercury amalgam fillings in the mother's teeth. These studies found that the mercury concentration in the urine of pregnant and lactating women positively correlated with the number of amalgam fillings and with frequency of fish consumption.

As a result, the German Federal Institute of Medicines has officially advised against the use of amalgam as a filling material during pregnancy and breastfeeding.

MERCURY IN YOUR MEDICINES

In spite of well-established health risks, organic mercurials are still added to prescription and non-prescription drugs, such as some medicines for haemorrhoids and skin infections.

Until recently, nearly all contact lens solutions contained ethyl mercury – otherwise called thimerosal or merthiolate – an organic mercurial used as an antibacterial agent. The ban on thimerosal in contact lens solutions did little to eliminate its use in other products, such as eardrops and nose drops. Thimerosal continues to be used today in a variety of health-related products; as a preservative for vaccines and other injections, cosmetics, and some drugs.

It is the thimerosal used in childhood vaccines that gives the greatest cause for concern. Investigators evaluating doses of mercury in the form of thimerosal used as a preservative in childhood immunisations found that they greatly exceeded US federal safety guidelines. The analysis showed increased risks for neurodevelopment disorders, autism and heart disease with increasing exposure to thimerosal in vaccines.

The epidemiological evidence is compelling and statistically conclusive. The prevalence of speech disorders, autism and heart disease was a function of the mercury dose that the children received. A fully vaccinated child in the US receives a whopping dose of over 230 micrograms of mercury from the vaccines. Could this be the cause of the modern epidemic of autism?

In today's world, mercury is no longer the messenger of the gods, but rather a man-made angel of death.

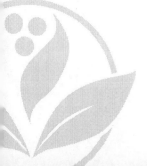

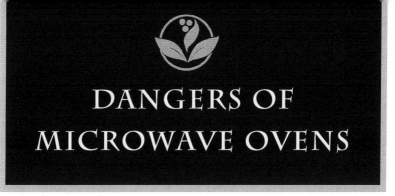

DANGERS OF MICROWAVE OVENS

When it comes to convenience, few devices can compare to the microwave. It is estimated that over 90 per cent of homes in North America have them. Are you among the millions of people every day exchanging your health for the convenience of microwave ovens? Before you use your microwave one more time, you might want to consider some facts.

The Germans invented the first microwaves and used them for preparing meals on a large scale during the invasion of Russia in World War II, thus eliminating the problem of cooking fuels. After the war, however, the Russians conducted thorough research on their biological effects. Alarmed by what they learned, the Russians banned microwave ovens in 1976.

WHAT IS WRONG WITH YOUR MICROWAVE?

Microwaves heat your food by causing it to resonate at very high frequencies. While this can effectively heat your food it also causes a change in the chemical structure of the food that can lead to health problems.

Heating food can cause problems by itself but when you heat it with microwaves you have the additional problem of the creation of negative frequencies that further devitalise your food. An illustration of the dangers posed by microwaves can be seen in a 1991 lawsuit involved a woman who had hip surgery and died because the blood used in her blood transfusion was warmed in a microwave. Blood is routinely warmed before transfusions, but not by microwave. The microwave altered the blood and it killed the woman.

MICROWAVES ALTER FOOD

By far, the most compelling evidence supporting the dangers of microwaves comes from a study done by Dr Hans Hertel, a Swiss food scientist, who concluded that microwave cooking significantly altered food's nutrients. This food, in turn, brought about changes in the body once ingested.

Dr Hertel's findings showed that microwave cooking resulted in significant and disturbing changes in the blood of individuals consuming microwaved milk and vegetables. Volunteers ate various combinations of the same foods cooked in different ways. All foods that were cooked through the microwave ovens caused changes in the blood of the volunteers. Haemoglobin levels decreased and overall white blood cell levels and cholesterol levels increased.

Microwave oven manufacturers insist that microwaved and irradiated foods do not have any significantly higher radiolytic (abnormal) compounds than do broiled, baked or other conventionally cooked foods. The scientific clinical evidence has shown that this is a lie.

The authorities seem more concerned with studies on what happens if the door on a microwave oven doesn't close properly. Their attention should be centred on what happens to food cooked inside a microwave oven. Since people eat this altered food, shouldn't there be concern for how altered molecules will affect our own human biological cell structure?

MICROWAVES ALTER NUTRITIONAL VALUE OF FOOD

Few people realise that many of the vitamins in food are rapidly destroyed by cooking. Even fewer know that microwaving destroys vitamins five times more quickly than regular cooking. Microwave heating, for example, inactivates vitamin B_{12}. After just six minutes of microwaving, nearly half of the vitamin B_{12} was destroyed when dietitians measured the levels after microwaving. Vitamin B_{12} was singled out for study since it is of vital importance in helping to prevent several major diseases that become more common as we grow older.

A study published in the November 2003 issue of the *Journal of the Science of Food and Agriculture* found that broccoli 'zapped' in the microwave with a little water lost up to 97 per cent of the beneficial antioxidant chemicals it contains. By comparison, steamed broccoli lost 11 per cent or fewer of its antioxidants.

Microwaves can cause uneven cooking

Microwaves do not cook food evenly. For example, frozen hamburgers, fish and warmed-up dishes all may have cool areas in them that could promote the growth of disease causing germs.

Microwaves release toxins in plastic containers

Do not heat food containing fat in a microwave using plastic containers because the combination of fat, high heat and plastics releases dioxins and other toxins into the food and ultimately into your cells. Dioxins are carcinogens and highly toxic.

Microwaves expose you to radiation

No one really knows what safe levels of exposure to microwave radiation are. Researchers have found that low-level exposure to microwave radiation can have cumulative effects on the eyes, resulting in cataracts. Experts also report a reduction in personnel efficiency, and even a possible link to cancer. Although the significance for humans of repeated exposure to low levels of microwave radiation is still unclear, there is enough evidence to warrant certain common sense precautions:

- Stay at least an arm's length away from an operating microwave oven.
- Do not operate an oven when it is empty.
- Do not operate an oven if the door will not close properly or is damaged in any way.
- Never tamper with the safety interlock switches or the fuse.
- Minimise the time of exposure to microwaves.

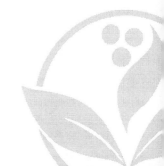

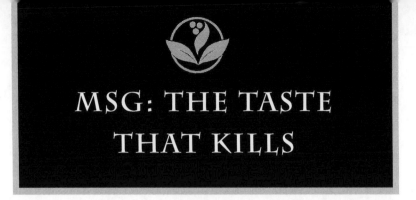

MSG: THE TASTE THAT KILLS

MSG (Mono Sodium Glutamate) is a food additive that enhances flavours in food. It really has no flavour of its own, but by stimulating your taste buds and nervous system, causes you to experience a more intense flavour from the foods that you eat.

Technically speaking, for food labelling purposes, MSG is approximately 78 per cent glutamic acid, 21 per cent sodium, and up to 1 per cent contaminants. However, the active ingredient, glutamic acid is present in smaller quantities in many, many foods without it being stated on their label.

To the food industry, it means increased profits, a simple way to balance and mask unwanted tastes in a product, and to make otherwise unpalatable foods acceptable. In particular, MSG helps replace flavour lost in many low-fat and no-fat foods.

To millions of consumers, however, it means exposure to the adverse effects from the additive and dangerous properties of this chemical.

The problem with MSG first came to the attention of doctors in 1968 when a Chinese physician, Dr Robert Ho Man Kwok, reported that he and his friends suffered numbness, weakness and palpitations when they dined in certain Chinese restaurants. The condition came to be known as the 'Chinese Restaurant Syndrome', and subsequent investigations indicated that Dr. Kwok's problem was a reaction to MSG, in particular the glutamic acid it contained.

GLUTAMIC ACID

It is unclear why some people have such a reaction to glutamic acid, but it may only become a problem when, in the manufacturing process, glutamic acid becomes free glutamate. When glutamate occurs naturally in vegetables, it doesn't seem to be harmful. However, when some people eat food containing MSG, they react immediately to the glutamate. Others do not react for at least 48 hours. Some reactions are dose related: the more you eat, the more reactions you will have. Some highly sensitive individuals will react when a very small amount is present in their food. Usually, the reaction will be the same and within the same period of time.

There has been an enormous amount of evidence linking the ingestion of free glutamate to serious health problems. These can extend far beyond the so-called 'Chinese Restaurant Syndrome'. The reactions usually involve different body systems, especially the brain. At the same time that glutamate is stimulating your taste buds, it is stimulating the entire nervous system as well because it is an excitotoxin.

THE A TO Z LIST OF POSSIBLE MSG PROBLEMS

ALS (amyotrophic lateral sclerosis, also known as Lou Gehrig's disease)
Alzheimer's disease-like symptoms

Anxiety attacks

Asthma-like symptoms

Attention Deficit Syndrome

Bloating

Burning sensations

Carpal Tunnel Syndrome

Chest pains

Depression

Diarrhoea

Disorientation and confusion

Dizziness

Drowsiness

Fatigue

Flushing

Gastric distress

Headaches and migraines

Hyperactivity in children

Infertility and other endocrine problems

Insomnia

Irregular or rapid heartbeat

Joint pain

Mood swings

Mouth lesions

Nausea

Numbness, for example, in the finger tips

Parkinson's disease

Seizures

Shortness of breath

Simple skin rash

Slurred speech

Stomach aches

Tremors

Vomiting

Weakness

In addition, some researchers believe that MSG can cause brain damage in children, and can affect how their nervous systems develop, so that in later years they may have learning or emotional difficulties.

Studies also indicate that women who ingest MSG while pregnant increase the risk of their developing foetus having smaller pituitary glands, thyroid glands, ovaries, or testes. This results in reproductive dysfunction in both females and males. MSG also increases the risk of developing sensitivities to numerous chemicals and other substances. It can certainly make you more sensitive to products containing aspartame.

WHAT TO DO

Avoiding glutamate is difficult since it is hard to identify in processed, packaged or restaurant food. Because foods now contain so many other chemicals, consumers find it more difficult to identify what substance in a food may be causing a reaction. Is it the glutamate, or the food itself, or the additives, or the pesticides?

It will be hard to tell until all the hidden sources are identified, but food manufacturers are doing a good job of keeping this ingredient hidden. One way to avoid the addition of free glutamate is by preparing your own food from fresh ingredients. Try to eliminate free glutamate from your diet for a few weeks and see how you feel. You may find it worth the effort.

The list of food products containing glutamate is growing. It is found in most salad dressing, processed meats, snack foods, soups, and prepared foods on the grocery store shelves. It is common in crackers, bread, frozen entrees, ice cream, frozen yogurt and low-fat foods. Be careful of the 'light' foods with reduced fat. Restaurants often add glutamate during preparation. Drinks, chewing gum, and candies are also potential sources.

Food is not the only source of glutamate. Soaps, shampoos, hair conditioners and cosmetics contain free glutamate, as well as binders for medication, nutrients and supplements.

Again we are confronted with how powerfully the things we put in our mouths can influence our health. It adds new meaning to the popular saying, 'You are what you eat'.

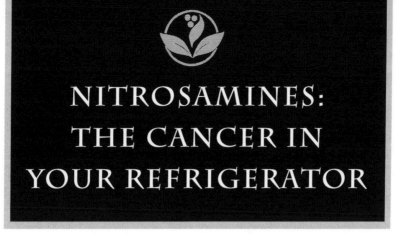

NITROSAMINES: THE CANCER IN YOUR REFRIGERATOR

There's a chemical that food manufacturers add to virtually all packaged meat products such as breakfast sausages, picnic hams, hot dogs, bacon, turkey bacon, bologna and many more. This chemical is used to give these meats a reddish colour so they still look fresh. By itself, this ingredient sounds completely harmless, but when you eat it, it forms other highly cancer forming chemicals known as **nitrosamines**.

Nitrosamines are a class of chemical compounds that were first described over 100 years ago. Approximately 300 of these compounds have been tested, and 90 per cent of them have been found to be cancer causing in a wide variety of experimental animals. Since nitrosamines are metabolised the same in humans and animals, it seems highly likely that nitrosamines are also carcinogenic in humans.

These nitrosamines are such powerful carcinogens that they are used in research to create cancer in laboratory animals. Clinical studies that monitored children who consumed this ingredient shockingly revealed a quadrupling of brain tumours and a 700 per cent increase in leukaemia.*

Another University of Hawaii study that tracked the dietary habits of nearly 200,000 people for seven years revealed that the consumption of processed meats containing this ingredient caused a whopping 6,700 per cent increase in pancreatic cancer.

Nitrosamines are so toxic that the USDA actually tried to ban them from all packaged meats in the 1970s, but the agency was overpowered by the corruption and influence of meat packing companies. So the ingredient is still legal to use, even though it is highly carcinogenic. When you eat this ingredient, it results in cancer-causing nitrosamines flowing through your entire digestive tract, ultimately promoting colon as well as pancreatic cancer.

SODIUM NITRITE

What's the name of this ingredient? Sodium nitrite. It is listed right on the label of almost every packaged meat product you can buy. If you own any bacon, sausage or luncheon meat product, check your refrigerator right now and see for yourself. You'll be amazed that this cancer-causing ingredient is in so many foods you've been buying for years!

The Safe Shopper's Bible (a nutrition handbook) explains that European countries banned the use of nitrite and nitrates in 1997 while the FDA has allowed their continued use in the USA. Jamaica seems to have followed the lead of the US in these matters.

Cured meats contain nitrosamines because sodium nitrite is added to cured meats as a preservative. Of all the cured meats, bacon has received the most attention. It almost always contains detectable levels of nitrosamines; possibly because the very high cooking temperatures used to fry bacon are conducive to nitrosamine formation.

Interestingly, though, since vitamin C and vitamin E inhibit nitrosamine formation, they are now being added to some cured meats. As a result of these strategies, there are now lower levels of nitrosamines in fried bacon and other cured meats than there were some years ago.

MAJOR SOURCES OF NITROSAMINES

These include:

- Fried bacon
- Cured meats
- Beer
- Nonfat milk powder
- Tobacco products
- Rubber products and rubber manufacturing
- Metal industries
- Pesticide production and use

- Certain cosmetics
- Certain chemical manufacturing

Nitrates can be found to some extent naturally in spinach, eggplant, beets, lettuce, turnip greens, green beans, radishes and celery. The nitrogen in chemical fertilisers oxidises into nitrates that these plants absorb. However, these vegetables are also rich in antioxidants, vitamins and minerals and this minimises nitrosamine formation. Organic vegetables have significantly less nitrates because of the natural compost used to fertilise the soil. Thus, nitrates in vegetables should not be used as an excuse not to eat them. It is, however, one more reason to choose organic products.

RECOMMENDATIONS

Here are some ways you can minimise your exposure to nitrosamines:

- Read food labels carefully. Avoid as much as possible, foods containing added sodium nitrite.

- Avoid very high cooking temperatures and frying as the very high heat used to cook many processed meats, like sausage and bacon, assist in the formation of nitrosamines.

- Use water filters as they can help eliminate nitrates and other unwanted chemicals from water.

- Use natural personal and skin care products as these do not contain chemical additives that can cause nitrosamine formation in the skin. I particularly recommend aloe-based products with added vitamins A, C and E.

- Practise good Cellular Nutrition with lots of antioxidant supplementation. Vitamins C and E, in particular, can help prevent nitrosamines from forming from the nitrates in your food.

- If you don't want to give up meats, eat only fresh organic and free-range chicken and turkey, and choose meats that do not have nitrates listed as one of the ingredients. Meats without nitrates are more perishable so eat them promptly or freeze them before the expiration date.

* Preston-Martin, S. et al. 'N-nitrosamine compounds and childhood brain tumors.' *Cancer Research* 42 (1982): 5240–5.

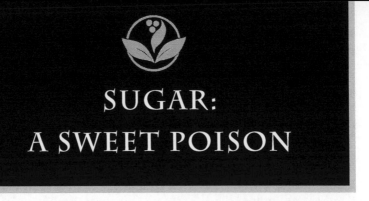

SUGAR:
A SWEET POISON

On average, each US citizen consumes an astounding two to three pounds of sugar each week. Sugar consumption has gone from only five pounds per year in 1900 to the current level of 135 pounds per person per year, and Jamaicans are closely following this trend.

This is not surprising as highly refined sugars in the forms of sucrose (table sugar), dextrose (corn sugar) and high-fructose corn syrup are being quietly processed into many popular foods such as bread, biscuits, breakfast cereals, mayonnaise, peanut butter, ketchup, spaghetti sauce, and a host of other convenience foods.

Heart disease and cancer were virtually unknown in the early 1900s but we now know that many of those modern ills may be related to our sweet tooth. Here is a list of some of the consequences of high sugar consumption. These are taken from a variety of medical journals and other scientific publications and are based on medical research.

SUGAR AND THE IMMUNE SYSTEM

In the 1970s, researchers found out that vitamin C was needed by white blood cells in high concentrations in order for them to destroy viruses and bacteria. Now, glucose and vitamin C both have similar chemical structures, and they compete with one another to enter the white blood cells. If there is excess glucose in the blood, there is going to be less vitamin C allowed into the cells. It doesn't take much: a blood sugar value of 120 mg/dl reduces the white blood cell function by 75 per cent. So when you eat sugar, be reminded that your immune system may be slowing down to a crawl.

Little wonder, therefore, that sugar greatly assists the uncontrolled growth of Candida (which causes yeast infections) while increasing your risk of infections from many bacteria, fungi and viruses.

A weak immune system will also make you more cancer prone. Sugar feeds cancer cells and has been connected with the development of cancer of the breast, ovaries, prostate, rectum, pancreas, lung, gall bladder and stomach. Sugar can impair the structure of your DNA and this will also influence your cancer risk.

SUGAR AND THE BRAIN

The consumption of refined sugars is associated with fluctuations in blood sugar levels – sometimes high, sometimes low. The brain is almost totally dependent on glucose (blood sugar) for its energy. Many nervous system disorders are related to (or made worse by) eating sugar and children are particularly at risk

These disorders include Attention Deficit Hyperactivity Disorder, depression, anxiety disorders, alcoholism and other addictions, epileptic seizures and migraine headaches. In juvenile rehabilitation camps, when children were put on a low sugar diet, there was a 44 per cent drop in antisocial behaviour.

Sugar can increase your risk of Alzheimer's disease and researchers have found that sugar intake is higher in people with Parkinson's disease.

SUGAR AND THE DIGESTIVE SYSTEM

Sugar can cause many problems with the gastrointestinal tract, including GERD (acid reflux disease), indigestion, malabsorption, ulcerative colitis and increased risk of Crohn's disease. Sugar can increase the size of your liver by increasing the amount of fat in the liver cells and creating fatty liver disease. Sugar can damage your pancreas and promote constipation. High sugar consumption will also increase your risk of gallstones and gall bladder disease.

SUGAR AND THE METABOLISM

Sugar has the potential to induce abnormal metabolic processes in a normal healthy individual and to promote chronic degenerative diseases.

Sugar, for instance, can cause a decrease in your insulin sensitivity, thereby causing abnormally high insulin levels and eventually diabetes. Sugar can also produce a significant rise in total cholesterol, triglycerides and bad cholesterol while decreasing your good cholesterol levels. It can also increase your risk of gout and is a major cause of obesity.

Sugar upsets the mineral relationships in your body: it causes chromium and copper deficiencies and interferes with the absorption of calcium and magnesium. It can cause hormonal imbalances such as increased oestrogen levels in men, elevated male hormones (androgens) in women (which exacerbates PMS) and decreased growth hormone levels. Sugar can result in fluid retention.

SUGAR AND PROTEINS IN THE BODY

Sugar can change the structure of protein and cause a permanent alteration in the way those proteins act in your body. Thus, by changing the structure of collagen (a protein in the skin) sugar can make skin age prematurely. By changing the proteins in the lens of the eye, sugar can cause cataracts. Diets high in sugar will increase free radicals and oxidative stress, known causes of accelerated ageing.

And the half has not been told. What about the effects of sugar on the heart, the blood pressure, the circulation, the blood vessels and your sex life? Don't allow a little sweet to make you really sour.

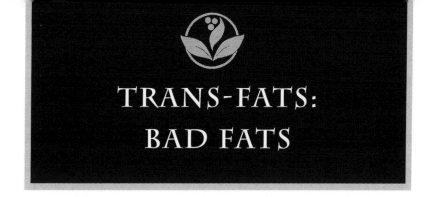

TRANS-FATS:
BAD FATS

Trans fatty acids, also known as trans-fats, are fats that are formed when vegetable oils are hardened into margarine or shortening. This process is called hydrogenation and involves bubbling hydrogen gas into various vegetable oils like corn, cottonseed or soybean oil. Because of this, trans-fats are also referred to as hydrogenated or partially hydrogenated fats.

Many food companies use trans-fats extensively instead of oil because it reduces cost, extends the storage life of products and can improve flavour and texture.

WHERE ARE TRANS-FATS FOUND?

Trans-fats are found in many other foods besides margarine and shortening, including fried foods like French fries and fried chicken, doughnuts, cookies, pastries and crackers. In the US, typical French fries have about 40 per cent trans fatty acids and many popular cookies and crackers contain between 30 and 50 per cent trans fatty acids. Doughnuts have about 35 to 40 per cent trans fatty acids.

While bakery items and fried foods are obvious sources of trans-fats, many other processed foods, such as cereals and waffles, can also contain trans-fats. One way to determine the presence of trans-fats in a food is to read the ingredient label and look for shortening, hydrogenated or partially hydrogenated oil. The higher up on the list these ingredients appear, the more trans-fats are present in the food.

One problem with trying to avoid trans-fats was that for a long time food companies were not required to list on nutrition labels how much trans-fats were in the food you were eating. Finally, in a step in the right direction, the

FDA in the US now requires food manufacturers to list trans-fats on Nutrition Facts labels. I hope the same regulation will soon be applied to Jamaican food manufacturers.

TRANS-FAT CONTENT OF MARGARINE, SHORTENING, AND VEGETABLE OILS

Food	Trans-Fat Content (%)
Stick Margarine	31
Tub Margarine	17
Diet Margarine	18
Vegetable Oil Shortening	20
Vegetable Salad Dressing	13

WHY ARE TRANS-FATS DANGEROUS?

Health authorities like the World Health Organization have expressed major concern over the levels of trans-fats in the modern diet. Medical research has shown that trans-fats have a host of negative effects on health.

On average, Americans consume about five grams of trans-fats per day, according to a 1999 study in the *Journal of the American Dietetic Association*. While that may sound tiny, research has linked even small amounts of trans-fats to an increased risk of heart disease. A 1994 Harvard University study found more than twice the risk of heart attacks among those who ate partially hydrogenated oils, which are high in trans-fats, compared with those who consumed little trans-fats.

Consuming trans-fats will:

- Increase the levels of bad cholesterol and promote heart disease and circulatory disorders.
- Increase the occurrence of several cancers.
- Depress the body's immune system.

- Decrease testosterone levels in men and increase abnormal sperm formation.

- Interfere with pregnancy, contribute to low birth weight in babies, and result in poor quality breast milk.

- Worsen diabetes, hypertension and obesity by increasing insulin resistance.

- Displace healthy fats, for example, the omega-3 fatty acids in fish oils, preventing them from performing their normal function.

- Disturb liver function.

In fact, several large studies in the US and elsewhere also show a strong link between premature death and consumption of foods high in trans fatty acids. It is calculated that trans fatty acids are responsible for about 30,000 premature deaths per year in the US.

A few food companies like Lipton, Cadbury and Nestle have taken steps to eliminate trans-fats from some of their products. In 2003, a lawsuit was filed in the US against Nabisco, the Kraft Foods company that makes Oreo cookies, seeking a ban on the sale of Oreo cookies because they contain trans-fats, making them dangerous to eat.

MY RECOMMENDATIONS

1. Have a balanced diet, high in fruit, vegetables and healthy low-fat protein.

2. Reduce your intake of processed fast foods, fried foods, cookies, cakes and crackers.

3. Carefully read the labels of processed foods and avoid those containing mostly hydrogenated or partially hydrogenated oils.

4. Cook primarily with olive oil, coconut oil or canola oil.

5. Supplement your diet with fibre, healthy omega-3 fats from fish oil and lots of antioxidant vitamins, minerals and herbs. These will help to reduce the negative impact of the trans-fats.

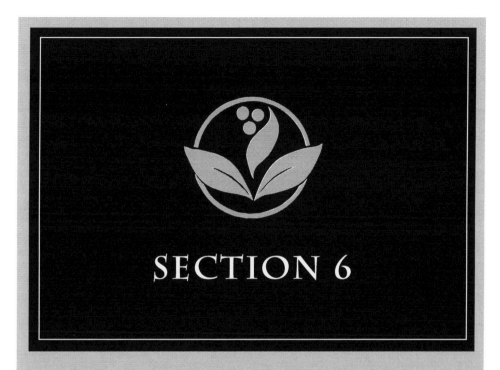

SECTION 6

WEIGHT
MANAGEMENT

*'Eat to live, and not live to eat. To lengthen
thy life, lessen thy means.'*

– Benjamin Franklin

www.anounceofprevention.org

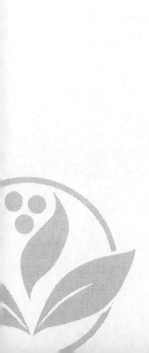

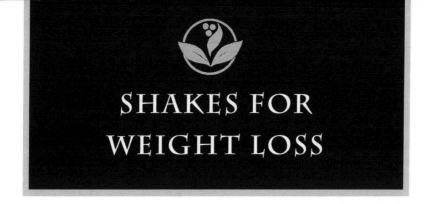

SHAKES FOR WEIGHT LOSS

M eal replacement supplements are one of the most popular food supplements available. As the name suggests, meal replacement supplements are meant to be eaten in place of regular meals. For over a quarter of a century, they have been used in weight loss programs. With the global epidemic of obesity and its related illnesses, medical research has focused on the use of meal replacement supplements for losing fat and maintaining optimal health. I myself have successfully used meal replacement supplements to assist thousands of my patients in successfully losing weight.

WHAT IS A MEAL REPLACEMENT SUPPLEMENT?

A meal replacement supplement is a portion-controlled meal in a drink, popularly called a shake. It usually contains less than 250 calories and is used to replace an entire meal. This helps you safely reduce your total calorie intake and thus lose weight. The shakes are usually low in fat and calories, but generous in healthy protein, various vitamins, minerals and fibre. High quality shakes are very nutrient dense and calorie poor and are really the healthiest fast food money can buy.

HOW EFFECTIVE ARE MEAL REPLACEMENTS?

A good answer comes from a study published in the *American Journal of Clinical Nutrition*. Researchers in Germany assessed the effects of a low-calorie diet using meal replacements on weight loss in a group of 100 obese patients.

Subjects were assigned to one of two groups. Group one consumed a low-calorie diet consisting of conventional foods. The second group used meal replacement drinks and snacks. Two years later, average weight loss in the group using the meal replacement supplements was *twice* as great compared to the group relying on conventional methods.

A second study presented at the North American Association for the Study of Obesity's annual meeting in Fort Lauderdale showed that people who followed a meal replacement plan for ten years weighed, on average, about 33 pounds less than people who didn't use a meal replacement plan.

This is one of the longest ever weight control studies to track how well people controlled their weight using meal replacement shakes. The results of these studies suggest that meal replacements are an effective weight-loss strategy in both the short and long term.

Approval ratings of meal replacements have been high, with very favourable scores for appetite satisfaction and taste.

HOW DO MEAL REPLACEMENTS WORK?

Meal replacements help people lose weight by providing a controlled number of calories and fats in a prefixed portion. They can simplify meal planning because they are convenient – easy to purchase, easy to store, and require little preparation. They are also reasonably priced, usually costing less than the meal they replace. Meal replacements reduce the number of decisions you have to make about what to eat and reduce your exposure to tempting foods that might result in overeating.

Most weight-loss programs that use meal replacement supplements recommend replacing two meals per day with shakes along with one regular meal to lose weight. Later, replacing only one meal per day will maintain weight. As an added bonus, reducing body fat results in a decreased risk of diabetes, high blood pressure, osteoarthritis and heart disease.

Using a meal replacement instead of an entire regular meal helps you to reduce your calorie and fat intake and control your blood sugar levels. If you are a diabetic using meal replacements, you will likely notice an immediate reduction in your blood sugar levels as you lose weight because you will be consuming fewer calories and fewer carbohydrates than you would with your usual meal. You should then check with your health care team about reducing the dosage of your diabetes medications or insulin.

WHAT ARE THE DRAWBACKS?

Not all meal replacement shakes are equal. Some popular brands are milk based and, in my opinion, contain far too much sugar. Some people find meal replacements boring and have feelings of deprivation. Again, selecting the right shake with appealing flavour and texture is necessary. High quality shakes offer various flavours with several recipes for making them interesting. I myself have used the meal replacement supplement produced by Herbalife International for the past 15 years and consider them the best shakes on the market today. Also, there are lots of books and websites (see Appendix) able to help you with creative ideas for improving satisfaction and variety in your diet while using meal replacements.

The strategy of using meal replacements works for as long as you stick with it. A support system, as provided by direct sales companies, ensures even better results from the use of their products.

Sample Menu Using Meal Replacement Supplements

Meal	Foods
Breakfast	Meal replacement shake
Snack	Fresh fruit / herbal tea / nuts
Lunch	Meal replacement shake
Snack	Fresh fruit / herbal tea / nuts
Dinner	4–6 ounces of fish or poultry (preferably organic)
	One small starch serving
	Three vegetable servings
	One salad serving
	One fruit serving
	One serving of soy milk

BOTTOM LINE

If you have trouble estimating portion sizes, find yourself eating too often or typically choose foods high in fat and calories, meal replacements would help you. We all know that losing weight is one thing, but keeping that weight off is a completely different story. Even using one meal replacement per day will help to keep weight from coming back.

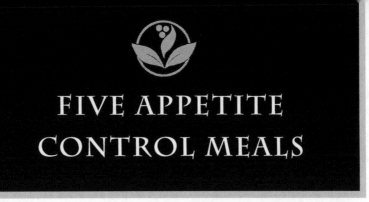

FIVE APPETITE CONTROL MEALS

More and more people are deciding to lose weight. Congratulations! But many fear that they may not be able to control their appetite and that hunger will spoil their weight loss program. The world's most successful weight control program (the one I use) is created by Herbalife International, and it is remarkably effective at appetite control.

However, as you lose weight, you may experience hunger at one time or another. There are several 'lifesaving' foods and beverages you can turn to when you are hungry that will not wreck your weight loss plan.

These foods and drinks are what I call **appetite-control foods**. What these foods and beverages have in common is that they make your stomach feel like it's full of rich foods. But in reality, you are filling up with foods that contain few calories or carbohydrates. Even though your stomach is full, you are not adding calories to your intake.

For example, if you eat one cup of peanuts versus a cup of shredded cabbage, your body can't really tell the difference for the first few minutes. Your stomach will turn off the hunger signals thinking you have eaten a large quantity of food regardless of whether you are eating cabbage or peanuts, but in fact the cabbage may only contain ten calories while the peanuts contain as many as 500 calories. Raw cabbage is, in fact, a great cure for stomach ulcers. But that's another article.

APPETITE CONTROL FOOD #1: FRESH, CLEAN WATER

That's right. Water is a powerful appetite suppressant and if you drink an 8-ounce glass of water when you first start feeling hungry, you will find that it suppresses your appetite in nearly every case. If you just drink a full glass of water and have the discipline to wait ten minutes, you will find that your appetite is either completely gone or dramatically reduced.

APPETITE CONTROL FOOD #2: GREEN TEA

Green tea, as distinct from black tea found in regular tea bags, is an excellent beverage for weight control. It not only controls appetite but it stimulates the body's metabolism to burn fat, enhances energy levels, offers protection from several cancers and is useful for hypertension and circulatory disorders. These benefits are not dependent on the small amount of natural caffeine found in green tea. Green tea can be had hot or cold with natural sweeteners.

APPETITE CONTROL FOOD #3: SOY PROTEIN SHAKES AND SNACKS

Soy protein shakes provide an excellent low calorie meal replacement drink that will satisfy your appetite. Here is a recipe for the shake I use and recommend to my patients. Combine eight ounces of unsweetened soy milk with two tablespoons of Herbalife Formula #1 protein powder and a slice of papaya, or half of a banana or apple, and blend. Avoid those popular meal replacement drinks that contain lots of sugar and carbohydrates and not enough protein. Roasted soy nuts, soy soups, fruit flavoured beverages and bars are other ways to use soy for appetite control while enjoying the many health benefits of soy.

APPETITE CONTROL FOOD #4: GREEN VEGETABLES

Vegetables such as lettuce, cabbage, bok choy, field greens and other leafy vegetables contain so few calories that you don't need to count them. Allow yourself to eat an unlimited quantity of any green leafy vegetable. They are 'free' foods that are rich in vitamins, minerals and cancer-fighting substances, and that fill your stomach and make you feel full, by turning off the hunger signals in your brain.

You can consume these green leafy vegetables in different ways. Most people don't like to eat them plain. Instead, you can make a salad and then add a low calorie salad dressing like homemade olive oil and vinegar. Avoid commercial salad dressings that boast of being low fat and cholesterol free. These may contain MSG, high-fructose corn syrup, and other unhealthy ingredients.

APPETITE CONTROL FOOD #5: APPLES

Eat the largest apple you can find of either the Jamaican or American variety. Sure, they contain some calories and some carbohydrates, but the apple will fill you up for quite a while, and that will stop you from eating far more calorie-rich foods.

Let me explain. If you are very hungry, it's very easy to reach for some processed foods like a bag of chips or crackers. You can start nibbling away until you've consumed 1000 calories or more. But, it's almost impossible to eat 1000 calories worth of apples. You'll probably fill up even before reaching 400 calories. Apples are great appetite suppressing foods because the fibre fills up your stomach and turns off your appetite before you overeat. The bonus is that apples contain various vitamins and minerals and anti-cancer agents.

OTHER NATURAL APPETITE SUPPRESSANTS

Fibre supplements

Swallow a couple of fibre tablets before you begin eating. Fibre tablets could include oat bran fibre, apple pectin fibre, or other natural fibres. Fibre creates a feeling of fullness with little food. Although several fibre supplements are available, I recommend one in which the fibre has been 'activated' to trap and eliminate any excess fat in your meal. Be careful to drink plenty of water as you take these tablets because without adequate water, they can slow up your digestive system. So, that's another reason to drink plenty of water.

Herbal tablets

A variety of herbs are effective at safely suppressing appetite and promoting weight loss. I recommend a tablet that contains a combination of several herbs (Ephedra free*) that suppress appetite while stimulating fat burning. They are far better than weight loss drugs.

---

*Ephedra is an ancient Chinese herb safely used for centuries to aid weight loss. Its use was recently banned in the US because of reported side effects from excessive use. This is unfortunate as this is a very useful herb when used properly.

'Have breakfast like a king, lunch like a prince, sup like a pauper.'
– Benjamin Franklin

Medical research now confirms the wisdom of generations of mothers, 'don't miss breakfast: it's the most important meal of the day'. Sadly, investigations indicate that in our modern societies as many as 20 per cent of people, including children, routinely miss this all-important meal. I suspect that this percentage may be even higher in Jamaica. In an effort to correct this, some societies have even instituted breakfast feeding programs in their schools.

WHY IS BREAKFAST SO IMPORTANT?

Eating breakfast is a vital step towards optimal health. Numerous scientific studies performed over the past 20 years have shown that there are many benefits to starting your day off with breakfast.

It improves your metabolism

The word breakfast itself indicates why this meal is so important: it literally means to break the fast. A fast is an extended period of time in which one goes without food. This occurs while we sleep at night. One way the body responds to fasting is to slow down the metabolism. So, the longer you go without food, the slower your metabolism becomes. Breakfast gets your metabolism going. Breakfast eaters tend to have higher metabolisms, and burn more calories to produce more energy.

It kick-starts your brain

Eating breakfast provides energy for the brain and improves alertness – very important for learning. Additionally, breakfast restores the body's blood sugar levels – the brain's energy source. Adults and children who eat breakfast have better concentration, memory, problem-solving abilities, mental performance, and mood than those who do not. After fasting overnight, eating a good breakfast ensures that our brains are fuelled and ready for work.

It powers up your day

Eating a nutritious breakfast gives your body the energy and nutrients it needs to get through the morning. We know that those who skip breakfast often don't make up for the missed nutrients later on in the day. A good breakfast can provide protein (for building and maintaining muscle), carbohydrates (for energy), fibre (for healthy digestive function), calcium (for building strong bones), iron (for healthy red blood cells and oxygen transport around the body), plus additional vitamins and minerals. These nutrients are essential for healthy growth and development.

It supports healthy weight control

When you miss breakfast, your body's general function (metabolism) slows down and remains low for the rest of the day. This makes it harder for your body to use up the energy from the foods you eat later in the day, possibly leading to weight gain. Also, without a healthy breakfast, we tend to get very hungry by mid morning and are more likely to fill up on snack foods that are convenient but poor in nutrients.

COMMON REASONS FOR SKIPPING BREAKFAST

In spite of the numerous benefits to eating breakfast, some people give a number of excuses for missing this very important meal. Some of these excuses are listed here.

1. **I don't have the time**

This is the number 1 reason people give for missing breakfast. Often, this results in a grab-and-go unhealthy breakfast or no breakfast at all. Still, according to the American Dietetic Association, 'breakfast doesn't have to be fancy or traditional to meet nutritional needs'. You can get started on simple, easy and healthy breakfasts.

2.   I am not hungry in the morning

This is a result of eating a full meal late in the evening or snacking late at night. When you go to bed with a full stomach, the body is still busy digesting all that food. Digestion goes into a slower gear during sleep and there is still food in the stomach in the morning. Your stomach needs a rest too. A tired stomach does not feel like having breakfast. Break that pattern by having the evening meal earlier and by having a digestible, nutritious breakfast.

3.   I am trying to lose weight

Many people skip breakfast in an effort to lose weight. Bad plan! As indicated earlier, skipping breakfast often leads to overeating later in the day. As a matter of fact, most obese people miss breakfast. It's easier to control one's weight by eating healthy smaller meals earlier in the day.

A SIMPLE SOLUTION

For over a decade, I have recommended a simple and nutritious liquid breakfast: I have a soy protein meal replacement shake along with an energising herbal tea blend. It's a fantastic combination that sets me up for a great day.

So, make an important health resolution – try my healthy breakfast every day for the next 30 days. You will feel the difference.

An important note: Many of those who do eat breakfast need to improve on their choices. According to Foodwatch, a US consulting firm, the number of people eating 'dessert for breakfast' – mainly refined carbohydrates in sugar filled processed cereals – is on the rise. These 'foods' make you fatigued and hungry by mid morning, so look for healthier alternatives.

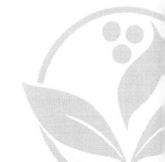

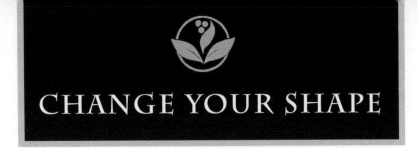

CHANGE YOUR SHAPE

As the epidemic of obesity escalates, medical experts are recognising that your body shape and body composition are even more important than your body weight. As individuals, we have our own unique shapes and we should recognise and appreciate that. But there is one area where the accumulation of excess fat is a medical disaster.

TRIM YOUR WAISTLINE

All the evidence points to excess upper body fat, what doctors call truncal obesity, as the most dangerous type of obesity. Men with a waist measurement greater than 39 inches, and women whose waists are more than 34 inches, have a 500 per cent increased risk of diabetes, high blood pressure, heart disease, cancer and a long list of other diseases.

A concentrated effort to trim the national waistline could empty half of Jamaica's hospital beds and dramatically reduce the pain and suffering created by the sicknesses listed above.

SHAPEWORKS

ShapeWorks is the latest, most scientifically sophisticated, yet easy-to-use plan designed to correct the problem of excess body fat. It was developed by Dr David Heber, the Director of the Center for Human Nutrition at UCLA. Dr Heber's new book *The LA Shape Diet* lays out clearly both the science and the practical elements of this approach to weight control. The program is based on four main concepts – The four **Ps**:

1. Personalise your program

In correcting obesity, one size does not fit all. Each body is unique in regard to lean body mass, body fat percentage and metabolic rate. With the appropriate equipment, we can now easily measure these indices on anyone and use this information to create a customised weight management program. Dr Heber has developed a simple tool that allows these calculations to be done even over the telephone.

2. **Plan your protein**

Your lean body mass (your non-fat weight) will tell you exactly the amount of protein you will need to consume each day in order to change your shape. The plan guides you in using healthy, convenient and economical protein foods to achieve your goal. Delicious soy protein based shakes are provided to make it easy for you to personalise your protein intake. Dr Heber has done extensive research to demonstrate that properly designed meal replacement shakes are extremely safe and effective for weight loss.

3. **Prioritise fruits and vegetables**

Health authorities are now recommending that we consume larger amounts of fruit and vegetables than ever before. For optimal health, men should eat nine and women seven servings of fruit and vegetables each day. Medical research continues to demonstrate that plants, especially fruit and vegetables, contain a large number of health enhancing substances. In ShapeWorks, fruits and vegetables are used creatively to facilitate healthy weight loss.

4. **Promote a healthy lifestyle**

ShapeWorks is not a quick fix scheme and it is essential to incorporate healthy lifestyle practices into the program. Particular attention should be paid to exercise and stress management, as these will greatly facilitate weight control while enhancing overall health and wellbeing.

With this in mind, the program has a built-in support system designed to provide all the necessary information, motivation and follow up. Hundreds of Jamaican ShapeWorks weight loss consultants have been trained and are now working all over the island. You can call us for a free body analysis and weight loss consultation or for information on how to contact a ShapeWorks consultant near you.

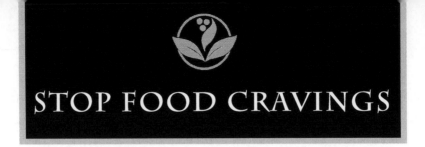

STOP FOOD CRAVINGS

Have you ever said to yourself, 'Why do I lose control of my eating? I am a successful person in other aspects of my life. But when it comes to eating, I am frustrated by my lack of will power and I am losing my self-esteem and placing my health at risk'. Well, the good news is that it may have nothing to do with a lack of willpower. Here are some common causes for those food cravings.

UNCONTROLLED BLOOD SUGAR

Research has confirmed that many of us simply cannot eat sugars and starches without it leading to food cravings. Unbalanced blood sugar levels are the major cause. You can check this out for yourself. Examine the highs and lows, the cravings created, and the physical, emotional and mental response you have to sugars and processed carbohydrates.

What happens to your blood sugar when you eat a high carbohydrate diet? It doesn't matter which processed carbohydrate foods you choose, carbohydrates break down into sugar (glucose) in your body and go into your blood. When you eat a high carbohydrate meal, your blood sugar levels can rise to a dangerous level.

Because your body cannot tolerate high blood sugar levels, it naturally produces the hormone insulin that takes sugar from the blood and deposits it into the cells. Large doses of insulin rush to the scene and clear out the sugar. As a result of this clearing, the opposite state occurs, called low blood sugar. You may be familiar with the feelings of low blood sugar – being tired, irritable, even shaky. To bring blood sugar levels back up, your body sends your brain a chemical message saying, 'I need sugar, eat sugar'. Hence you crave sodas, bread, biscuits, cakes, pasta, or anything with sugar or starch. In effect, carbohydrate cravings are a biochemical response to low blood sugar.

ALCOHOL: A POISON

Biochemically sugar and alcohol are the same. The alcohol and the sweets both send your blood sugar high but the alcohol is able to spike your blood sugar twice as quickly. In addition, alcohol contains empty calories – calories without any nutritional value. Alcohol is also toxic to your brain. A single drink will destroy as many as 100,000 brain cells. So, if you have carbohydrate cravings, stop taking alcohol.

BRAIN MALNUTRITION

For some people, compulsive eating is related to deficiencies in brain chemicals called neurotransmitters. If you lack these substances – serotonin, dopamine, or one of the other essential chemical communicators in your brain – the resulting response is a craving for carbohydrates, especially sugar and bread products. Because of the high sugar content of foods like flour products, chocolates, potatoes, white rice and corn, many people compulsively eat them when these deficiencies exist. Increasing your intake of healthy, high quality protein like soy or fish will diminish those cravings.

EMOTIONAL DISTURBANCES

Food cravings may also result from emotional disturbances. Feelings of emptiness, deprivation or lack of love and support may cause the individual to seek comfort and satisfaction in food. Overeating may certainly be a manifestation of depression.

Bulimia is a very serious eating disorder in which the individual overeats and then induces vomiting and purging to allow them to eat more. This disease needs expert medical attention.

THE SOLUTION

If you are ready to put an end to your food cravings and overeating, here are a few simple guidelines.

1. **Eat enough healthy protein**

Each person has a level of protein in their daily diet that is right for them. Experts recommend that you eat 1 gram of protein for each pound of your lean body mass. Adequate protein will prevent blood sugar imbalance.

2. Eat healthy carbohydrates

Make fresh fruit and vegetables your main carbohydrate foods. It is recommended that women eat seven servings and men nine servings of fresh fruits and vegetables on a daily basis. These foods are excellent sources of fibre, vitamins, minerals, antioxidants and cancer protective substances.

3. Eat five or more times daily

Do not go for long periods without eating. Between your main meals, have a few healthy snacks – healthy protein, fruit or vegetables.

4. Take supplements

Have a high quality multivitamin and mineral supplement with each main meal. Vitamins and minerals are essential for proper blood sugar control and healthy brain chemistry.

5. Get support

Find a support system that will assist you in following the guidelines above as well as providing the caring and emotional support you may need.

 Control your food. Don't let your food control you.

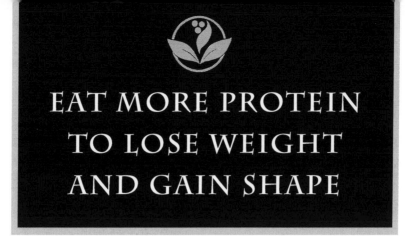

EAT MORE PROTEIN TO LOSE WEIGHT AND GAIN SHAPE

There are three main groups of foods. These are proteins, carbohydrates and fats. All three are important. A number of recent weight loss diets focus on the fact that it is not just how much you eat that creates excess fat, but very importantly, the proportions of these three food groups, particularly protein, in your diet. Unfortunately, many of these diets are not based on the most recent scientific information. Let us look at the facts about protein and weight loss.

WHY IS PROTEIN IMPORTANT?

Protein is made up of units called amino acids, some of which our bodies cannot manufacture and which must be obtained from our food. Protein is essential for building and maintaining muscles, as well as repairing the muscle damage that occurs during exercise. Protein is also needed to make red blood cells, produce hormones, boost your immune system (which fights disease), and help keep hair, fingernails and skin healthy. Individuals who are protein deficient may complain about having hair that falls out easily and fingernails that grow slowly and break easily. A low protein diet may create hormonal imbalances and women who eat a protein-poor diet may even stop having menstrual periods.

HOW CAN PROTEIN BURN FAT?

Carbohydrates are the primary energy foods that are converted into blood sugar (glucose) in the body. However, if we eat more carbohydrates than we need, the excess is stored in the body as fat, usually around the waistline. You can get very fat from eating carbohydrates even if you have no fat in your diet. If you restrict your intake of carbohydrates, then your body will begin burning up excess body fat as the alternative source of energy. One major reason for this is that a low carbohydrate diet will lower the levels of the hormone insulin in the blood. Carbohydrate foods increase the body's production of insulin which causes excess calories to be stored as fat. Protein foods tend not to stimulate insulin production, thereby encouraging the body to burn fat instead of storing it.

HEALTHY PROTEIN

More protein does not mean more meat, and unlike the Atkins dietary approach, I do not recommend eating lots of animal fats. Those fats are very saturated (that is, they contain the least healthy fats) and are also heavily contaminated with chemicals like hormones and pesticides.

Whereas high meat consumption can be burdensome to the kidneys, soy protein has been repeatedly shown to enhance kidney function. In addition, soy is good for the heart, the circulation, cholesterol levels, hormonal balance and bone health as well as being protective against many cancers.

Soy is my preferred protein. It is a very tasty food product, and it is available in the weight and health management programs I use. Other sources of high quality protein are whey, fish, organic poultry and eggs, beans, peas and nuts.

PRINCIPLES OF HIGH PROTEIN WEIGHT LOSS

There are two main principles that govern this approach to weight and shape management:

1. **Customise your protein intake**

Each person has an optimal healthy level of protein consumption. This is based on their lean body mass. The formula is 1 gram of protein daily for each pound of lean body mass. Dietitians have simple instruments to do this calculation for you.

2. **Eat healthy carbohydrates**

Most of your carbohydrates should come from fruits and vegetables. The formula is seven servings daily for women and nine servings daily for men of fruit and vegetables. One medium sized fruit or half a cup of vegetables constitutes a serving.

Benefits of a Healthy Program

I have often mentioned the Cellular Nutrition Program for optimal nutrition. Well, this plan incorporates those principles while allowing you to enjoy the extraordinary benefits of protein in a healthy, convenient way.

- Successful weight loss, even for the chronically obese.

- Shape management resulting in selective fat loss, especially from the abdomen, without muscle loss.

- Significant improvement in the control of blood sugar, blood pressure, cholesterol and triglyceride levels.

- Appetite control with increased energy and freedom from hunger.

- General health benefits from Cellular Nutrition.

- High fibre and phytonutrient intake from the vegetables and fruits.

- Improved water consumption because fruits and vegetables are water-rich foods.

- The program includes balanced supplementation of vitamins and minerals to ensure optimal Cellular Nutrition.

- When weight loss is achieved, the program can be modified for weight and health maintenance.

So, control your carbs, control your insulin, control your fat.

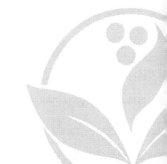

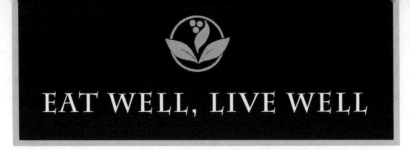

EAT WELL, LIVE WELL

The modern food industry spends billions of advertising dollars annually in brainwashing us into unhealthy patterns of eating. The current epidemic of chronic diseases and obesity is, in large measure, a reflection of these unhealthy eating habits. We are indeed 'digging our graves with our teeth'.

But it is not just what you eat, but also how you eat that is important. Here are some tips on eating well.

LISTEN TO YOUR BODY

Learn to listen to the signals your body sends you. The rule is very simple: eat when you are truly hungry and stop when you are satisfied. Use food to feed your body and not your emotions. From the time we were infants we associated food with safety, security and love. The breast or the bottle was used to comfort us whenever we were distressed either physically or emotionally. Naturally, as adults we still try to satisfy our need for love or to relieve our stress and anxiety with food.

Many people eat because they think it is time to eat, not because their body needs food. This encourages overeating. Start listening to your body. Do not overeat. The advice of my uncle of blessed memory is still applicable: 'Son, always leave the table feeling that you could have had a little bit more'.

PAY ATTENTION TO THE FOOD

Try to focus fully on the process of eating your meal. Many of us are accustomed to eating while watching television, conducting business or reading the newspapers. This robs you of your awareness of what you are doing so you will often unconsciously overeat because you have missed the signals that your body has had enough food. To prevent this, do the following things.

- Eat in a relaxed environment with minimal distractions. Before you begin eating take a few deep breaths, relax your body and give thanks for the gift of food that has been provided for your body.

- Chew your food until it is liquid, or almost liquid, in your mouth before swallowing. Become aware of the flavour, texture and the sensations that you experience from the food in your mouth.

- Do not put the next bite of food into your mouth until you have swallowed the previous one. Try setting down your knife and fork and relaxing between mouthfuls instead of busily piling food onto your fork or spoon. Take time to fully enjoy each bite.

EAT AT THE RIGHT TIME

When you eat is very important. Do not put the next meal into your stomach until you have digested the previous one (usually at least three hours after eating). For most of us, a nutritious soy based protein shake with or without some fresh fruit is an excellent choice for breakfast. Your digestive power is greatest at midday when your body secretes more stomach acid, bile and digestive enzymes. Until fairly recently in our history, most people ate their main meal in the middle of the day with a lighter meal in the evening. Eating more at lunch and less at dinner can improve digestion and enhance sleep.

Do not eat and then lounge or lie down immediately. Allow at least two hours after your last meal before going to bed.

TAKE SUPPLEMENTS

Modern medicine has finally agreed that the modern food supply is not providing us with all the nutrients we need for optimal health. The American Medical Association itself now recommends that everyone should take vitamin and mineral supplements daily.

For over a decade, I have supplemented my diet on a daily basis with a nutritional plan called the Cellular Nutrition Program. I have also recommended it to thousands of people with some remarkable results. I suggest that you find a good program (not a random collection of different vitamins) and begin the habit of taking daily supplements now.

If you wish to live well, then please start to eat well.

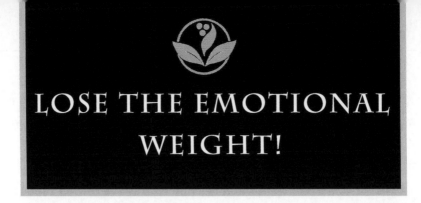

LOSE THE EMOTIONAL WEIGHT!

Although there are many different programs for losing weight, most do not achieve lasting results because they may not address all the underlying factors that led to the problem in the first place.

For many overweight individuals, the unhealthy relationship that they have with food is in fact a mirror of unhealthy relationships in other areas of their lives, especially the relationship that they have with themselves. Let's highlight some of these poor food relationships.

SUBSTITUTING FOOD FOR LOVE

Many of us learnt as children to associate food with love and reward. Common scenarios like, 'Be a good girl and Mom will give you a candy' or 'If you don't behave yourself, I won't give you any ice cream tonight' are innocently repeated admonitions by well meaning parents all over the world. The child quickly learns to associate certain foods with pleasure and satisfaction. Small wonder that as adults we use those foods to soothe our feelings of depression and loneliness.

Experts have identified so-called comfort foods – foods that we use to make us feel good. These foods have the ability to increase the levels of certain pleasure promoting chemicals, like serotonin, in the brain cells. Chocolates, ice cream and some other confectionaries head the list of pleasure foods.

GETTING FAT TO FEEL SAFE

Some people actually seek security in being big and fat. For some, their actual large size gives them a feeling of power and security that they even use, sometimes, to intimidate others.

For others, the fat can be a form of cocoon or shield or repellant. A number of women, for example, who have experienced sexual abuse become obese because, at a subconscious level, they are trying to look unattractive as a means of reducing the risk of future assault.

ABUSING YOURSELF WITH FOOD

There are those who suffer from low self-esteem, guilt and shame and who find ways to self-destruct and self-abuse. Food becomes a convenient and effective weapon in this instance. This syndrome can take on many forms ranging from disfiguring obesity and binge eating (with subsequent purging and/or vomiting) to the other extreme, anorexia nervosa where individuals literally starve themselves, sometimes to death.

ADDICTION TO FOOD

Some people have addictive personalities. The same factors that can create an addiction to alcohol, cigarettes, cocaine or sleeping tablets can also cause an addiction to food. But, because eating is so socially acceptable, this a ddiction often goes undetected for a long time until morbid obesity becomes manifest.

THE IDEAL WEIGHT LOSS PROGRAM

Because of the above issues, the ideal weight loss program should not only be safe, effective, convenient and nutritionally sound, but it should have a built in support system.

The data clearly shows that the most successful weight loss programs are those that provide their clients with ongoing person to person instruction, follow-up and emotional support.

The weight loss programs and products I have successfully used on thousands of clients have demonstrated the effectiveness of this approach. Conventional medical dietary approaches to weight loss have had an abysmal 90 per cent failure rate. In the hands of trained lay nutritional consultants, our programs at the Vendryes Wellness Centre have approached a 90 per cent success rate. You really have no reason for not starting your before Christmas weight loss program today.

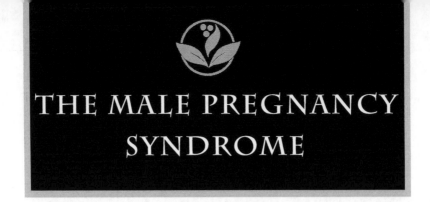

THE MALE PREGNANCY
SYNDROME

It is a common sight to see men whose swollen bellies make them look pregnant. They have what I call the male pregnancy syndrome. This condition is associated with a high incidence of diabetes, hypertension, heart disease, circulatory problems and metabolic disorders, like high levels of cholesterol, triglycerides and uric acid in the blood. Other seemingly unrelated conditions like chronic fatigue, erectile dysfunction, snoring and sleep apnea are also related to this kind of obesity. Medical research suggests that a man with a waist measurement of over 39 inches will increase his risk of diabetes, high blood pressure and heart disease by over 500 per cent!

THE FACTS

Here are some facts about the male pregnancy syndrome:

- The obesity of the male pregnancy syndrome involves an accumulation of fat on the upper trunk – from the neck to the abdomen – often without the arms, legs or buttocks being involved. This is known as 'apple' shaped or truncal obesity. We also know it as 'beer belly' or 'big gut'.

- This 'pregnancy' fat is not just under the skin. It accumulates inside the abdominal cavity, covering and infiltrating the internal organs and is associated with the serious medical conditions mentioned above. The liver is particularly prone to be strangled by this fat, creating a condition called fatty liver. Hormonal imbalance, with high levels of female hormones, often develops leading to sexual dysfunction.

- Of course, women who are not truly pregnant can also develop this apple-type obesity. Their buttocks, legs and arms may be normal but they display the large abdomen of male pregnancy sometimes accompanied by large breasts and neck. They carry the same risks as their male pregnancy counterparts.

Pear shaped obesity is more common in women, with fat accumulation in the lower abdomen, thighs and buttocks, most of it located beneath the skin. This kind of fat is less active metabolically and represents stored excess calories. This is a less dangerous pattern of obesity and is associated with fewer medical problems.

- After cigarette smoking, obesity remains the most common preventable cause of death in the world today. Male pregnancy type obesity is a particularly common, dangerous, preventable and correctable condition.

THE SOLUTION

The usual recommendation to lose weight by just cutting back on food consumption is often inadequate in dealing with this kind of obesity. The individual may lose some weight from their arms, legs, neck and face but relatively little from the abdomen. What, therefore, is the best way to deal with this male pregnancy syndrome?

- A highly effective approach is a program I use called ShapeWorks. Much of the epidemic of abdominal obesity is due to the over consumption of carbohydrates, especially simple and refined sugars and starches. The ShapeWorks plan deprives the body of excess carbohydrates causing the system to burn the fat stored in the abdomen. This program focuses on fat loss rather than just weight loss. It helps you reshape and contour your body while retaining your muscle mass.

- The ShapeWorks weight loss consultants at the Vendryes Wellness Centre are equipped to do a body analysis which calculates your percentage of body fat and your ideal body weight. Based on this information, the program is then customised to suit your needs. This is the most scientific and effective way I know for healthy fat reduction.

- Protein, vitamin and mineral supplements should be added to your diet to ensure balanced Cellular Nutrition. Keen attention must also be paid to a generous intake of water and fibre.

- Abdominal exercises alone are not effective in dealing with male pregnancy. Make nutritional changes your first priority. Then, I recommend 30 minutes or more of brisk walking, three to five times weekly depending on your fitness level. A more comprehensive exercise program can then be gradually introduced.

Let us all make a commitment to reduce this major health risk in our society – Male Pregnancy. One of our consultants would be happy to offer you a free consultation.

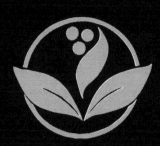

APPENDICES

- Low Carbohydrate Diet Sheet

- General Diet Sheet

- Cancer Diet Sheet

- Use of Natural Progesterone Cream

- The Barnes Test for Thyroid Function

- Estrogen Dominance /Progesterone Deficiency Questionaire

- Low Thyroid (Hypothyroidism) Questionaire

- Candida (Yeast) Overgrowth Questionaire

- Low Testosterone Questionaire

'Do not follow where the path may lead.
Go instead where there is no path and leave a trail.'

www.anounceofprevention.org

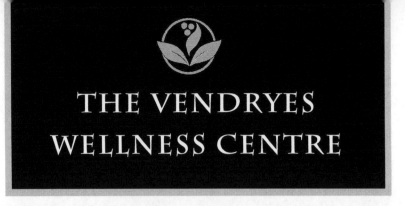

THE VENDRYES WELLNESS CENTRE

HIGH PROTEIN/ LOW CARBOHYDRATE DIET SHEET

Proteins	Complex Carbohydrates	Vegetables
Soy Protein Shake Drinks	Sweet Potato	Broccoli, Cauliflower, Cabbage, Brussel Sprouts
Fresh Fish	Yam, Green Banana (1)	Asparagus
Sardines in Water or in Sardine Oil	Squash, Pumpkin	Lettuce, Spinach, Callaloo
Cod Fish – Desalted	Steamed Brown Rice	Carrots – Raw or Steamed
Salmon or Tuna	Steamed Basmati Rice	Green Beans and Peas
Unsalted Mackerel	Whole Wheat Pasta	Cucumber, Zucchini
Skinned Chicken Breast (Organic)	Oatmeal or Barley	Green Peppers, Okra
Tofu / Bean Curd	Whole Grain Bread (not Brown) – 1 slice only	Mushrooms
Textured Vegetable Protein	Beans/Peas/Nuts	Onion and Garlic
Organic Eggs (Whites Preferred)	Corn ½ – Boiled or Roasted	Tomato, Red Pepper
Low-Fat Cottage Cheese	Strawberries, Cranberries	Watercress, Celery
Skinned Turkey Breast	Watermelon or Cantaloupe	Artichoke
Veggie Burger, Veggie Chunks or Steaks	Apples (Local or American)	Cho-cho
Bean Soup and stews	Small Orange or ½ Grapefruit	
Soy Milk, Nuts, Cheese	Pineapple – small slice	
Rice Milk and Miso Soup	Papaya – small slice	

- For each meal, choose one portion of protein, half a portion or less of carbohydrates and 2 portions or more of vegetables.
- One portion is the approximate size of your fist, or the amount that would cover the palm of your hand.

Additional Instructions
Snacks allowed – protein bars, soy nuts, protein drinks, raw vegetables and nuts may be eaten between meals. Avoid high carbohydrate snacks especially those with sugar, flour and starches.

GENERAL DIET SHEET

Foods You Can Eat Daily	Foods You Can Eat 3 to 4 Times Per Week	Foods You Avoid
Fresh Fruits	Organic Eggs	White Rice
Raw Vegetables/Salads	Whole Wheat Flour	Fried, Jerked Foods
Lightly Steamed or Stir Fried Vegetables	Sardines in Spring Water or Sardine Oil	White Sugar
Soy Products e.g. Shakes, Veggie Meats, Soy Milk, Soy Cheese, Tofu, Miso, Tempeh	Avocado Pears	Dairy Products – Milk, Butter, Cheese, Ice Cream
Green Banana, (1 per serving) Irish or Sweet Potatoes (small portion)	Organic Chicken (Skinned)	White Flour Products (for example, Dumplings, White Bread, Crackers, Cakes, Buns)
Fish – Baked or Steamed	Organic Turkey Breast	Highly Processed Foods
Pumpkins, Squash, Yellow Vegetables	Nuts – Peanuts, Cashews, Almonds	Gravies, Oils, Fats
Porridge – Bran/Oats	Olive Oil or Coconut Oil	Canned Meats
Unprocessed Cereals	Cornmeal/Barley/Oats	Canned Drinks
Brown Rice	Curries	Soft Drinks and Diet Sodas
Yams (small portion)	Whole Grain Bread (not Brown)	Red Meats, Pork, Non-organic Chicken
Coconut Water	Honey	Sugar Substitutes – Aspartame, etc.
Vegetable/Bean/Pea Soup	Corn on the Cob	Hydrogenated Vegetable Oils, Margarine
Beans/Peas/Nuts/Seeds	Ackee & Salt Fish	Shell Fish – Crab, Lobster, Shrimps
Fresh Fruit, Vegetables and Green Juices	Soy Ice Cream	Organ Meats – Liver, Kidney
Dried or Blended Fruit		

• Aim to have some live (uncooked) food included in every meal.

• Schedule regular meal times. Sit down and focus on paying attention to your eating.

• Eat slowly and chew the food thoroughly.

CANCER DIET SHEET

Foods You Eat	Foods You Avoid
Fresh Organic Vegetables & Juices – emphasise the following groups **Cruciferous Vegetables:** Cauliflower, Brussels Sprouts, Broccoli, Cabbage.	**Foods High in Saturated Fats:** Beef, Sausages, Pork, Ham, Tinned Meats, Cream, Lard etc.
Green Leafy Vegetables: Callaloo, Carrot Tops, Kale, Dark Lettuce, Watercress and Spinach.	**Refined Oils:** Peanut, Corn, Soybean, Sunflower, Margarines. Use only cold-pressed, virgin or unrefined oils.
Root Vegetables: Beets, Carrots, Radishes, Japanese Radishes (Daikon), Sweet Potatoes, Turnips, Yams and Asparagus.	**Foods cooked in the following ways:** Jerked, Barbecued, Fried or Roasted.
Fresh Organic Fruits: Apples – Jamaican and American, Papayas, Pineapple and Honeydew Melon, Apricots, Guava, Peaches, Plums, Prunes, Currants, Kiwi, Blackberries, Cranberries, Gooseberries and Elderberries. Also Apricot Kernels (3–6 per day)	**Stimulants:** Coffee, Black Tea, Alcohol, Canned and Carbonated Beverages.
Sprouted and Cooked Cereals: Brown Rice, Millet, Rye, Barley, Buckwheat, Corn and Oats. Sprouted Wheat Grass and Barley Grass Juices	**All Unsafe Preservatives** and Food Colourings (read labels).
Seafood if advised: younger, faster swimming fish. Sardines are preferable. Avoid shellfish.	**Foods Cooked in Aluminum** Cookware or with Aluminum Utensils (Use stainless steel, ceramic or glassware).

Cancer Diet Sheet continues

Foods You eat	Foods You Avoid
Vegetable Protein: Legumes include Lentils (as Sprouts), Chickpeas, Kidney Beans, Lima Beans, Green Peas (Split Peas) and Mung Beans (as Sprouts). Nuts (except peanuts) and Seeds are okay.	**Microwaved Foods** (which change many amino acids into an unstable form, and promote free-radical production).
Other Proteins: For some patients, organically produced poultry in moderation, on an occasional basis. Live Yogurt, Organic Buttermilk and Low-fat Cottage Cheese if acceptable on a limited basis.	**Wheat Flour Products:** Bread, Biscuits, Buns, Cakes, Pastry.
Supplemental Plant Foods: (1) Sea-vegetable Salads, which may include Dulse, Kelp, Hiziki, Kombu and Alaria. (2) Generous seasoning of dishes with fresh Garlic and fresh Ginger everyday; (3) Light seasoning with Turmeric (1gram daily), Cumin Seeds and fresh Basil. (4) Liberal use of Shitake, Reishi and Maitake Mushrooms and Chinese or Japanese Green Tea everyday.	**Dairy Products:** Cow's Milk, Butter, Cheese. **Sugar of all types:** Honey, Jams, Soft Drinks, Fruit Juices, Chocolate, and Ice-cream
Fats: Use only Cold-pressed (usually labeled as unrefined) Olive and Linseed Oils, and unrefined Coconut Oil.	**Trans-Fats:** Look for the words *hydrogenated or partially hydrogenated* on food labels.

INSTRUCTIONS FOR THE USE OF
NATURAL PROGESTERONE CREAM

1. Select the right cream. Read the label carefully. The ideal type of cream should be labeled Natural Progesterone Cream USP 2% or 4%. Avoid creams that claim to contain natural progesterone but which actually contain progestin drugs. Avoid using progesterone creams that also contain oestrogen or herbs with oestrogen-like activity.

2. Apply the cream twice daily to the wrists, inner arms, inner thighs or neck; vary the site of application from day to day. Absorption is optimal from skin that is soft, with underlying veins or muscles near the surface. Skin over fatty tissues absorbs the cream more slowly. Do not wash or apply anything else to the area for 30 minutes after applying the natural progesterone cream.

3. If menstruating, count the first day of the menstrual period as day one. Apply __ teaspoonful __ times daily to the skin from day 8 to day 28 of your monthly cycle. The label will indicate the recommended quantity depending on the strength of the cream.

4. If not menstruating, apply the natural progesterone cream using the same routine as above for 14 days and rest for 14 days, each month i.e. 14 days on and 14 days off.

5. It is advisable that you consult a health care provider familiar with the use of natural progesterone cream to monitor your treatment.

THE BARNES TEST FOR THYROID FUNCTION

Name: .... Sex: .... Age: ....

1. The night before the test, shake down the thermometer and place it by your bedside. A mercury thermometer is more desirable than a digital one.

2. On awakening in the morning before doing anything, place the t hermometer snugly under the armpit and leave it there for ten minutes by the clock. Remain quietly in bed during that period.

3. Remove the thermometer and record the temperature reading. Repeat the test for 5 or more days.

Men, girls before onset of menstruation and women after menopause may do the test on any day of the month. Women during their menstruating years should ideally start the test on the second or third day after the start of their period.

Readings below the normal range of 97.8 to 98.2° F (36.55 to 36.78° C) strongly suggests low thyroid function. Readings above the range may suggest infection or an overactive thyroid gland.

Date	Temperature	Notes

ESTROGEN DOMINANCE /PROGESTERONE DEFICIENCY QUESTIONAIRE

Read each question carefully and check if it applies to you. When you finish, calculate your score.

1. Do you have premenstrual breast tenderness? ☐
2. Do you have premenstrual mood swings? ☐
3. Do you have premenstrual fluid retention? ☐
4. Do you have premenstrual headaches? ☐
5. Do you have migraine headaches? ☐
6. Do you have severe menstrual cramps? ☐
7. Do you have heavy periods with clotting? ☐
8. Do you have irregular menstrual cycles? ☐
9. Do you have uterine fibroids? ☐
10. Do you have fibrocystic breast disease? ☐
11. Do you have endometriosis? ☐
12. Have you been diagnosed with breast or uterine cancer? ☐
13. Have you had problems with infertility? ☐
14. Have you had more than one miscarriage? ☐
15. Do you have joint pain? ☐
16. Do you have muscle pain? ☐
17. Do you have decreased libido? ☐
18. Have you been gaining weight? ☐
19. Do you have anxiety or panic attacks? ☐
20. Have you had seizures? ☐

Total Score – Add up your 'yes' answers

1–5   – Estrogen dominance is unlikely
5–10   – Estrogen dominance is possible
10–15 – Estrogen dominance is probable
15–20 – Estrogen dominance is very likely

LOW THYROID (HYPOTHYROIDISM)
QUESTIONAIRE

Read each question carefully and check if it applies to you. When you finish, calculate your score.

1.   Do you have fatigue or low energy levels?   ☐
2.   Do you find it hard to concentrate?   ☐
3.   Do you have poor short term memory?   ☐
4.   Do you have depressed moods?   ☐
5.   Do you have dry skin?   ☐
6.   Are you sensitive to the cold?   ☐
7.   Does your resting body temperature run below the normal 98.6°?   ☐
8.   Do you have cold hands and feet?   ☐
9.   Do you have decreased sweating?   ☐
10.   Are you having hair loss or thinning hair?   ☐
11.   Do you have decreased body hair?   ☐
12.   Do you have thinning or loss of your eyebrows or eyelashes?   ☐
13.   Do you have elevated cholesterol?   ☐
14.   Do you have less than one bowel movement a day?   ☐
15.   Do you have difficulty losing weight?   ☐
16.   Do you have a slow pulse?   ☐
17.   Do you have low blood pressure?   ☐
18.   Do you have fluid retention?   ☐
19.   Have you had problems with infertility or miscarriages?   ☐
20.   Do you have recurrent infections?   ☐

Total Score – Add up the number of 'yes' answers

< 10   – It is not likely that you have low thyroid function
11–15   – Low thyroid function is a definite possibility
> 15   – Low thyroid function is very likely

CANDIDA (YEAST) OVERGROWTH
QUESTIONAIRE

Read each question carefully and check if it applies to you. When you finish calculate your score.

1. Do you have recurrent vaginal yeast infections? ☐

2. Do you have athlete's foot? ☐

3. Do you have jock itch? ☐

4. Do you have rectal itching? ☐

5. Do you have fungal infections under the toenails or fingernails? ☐

6. Have you taken antibiotics multiple times during your life? ☐

7. Do you have abdominal bloating, cramping or gas? ☐

8. Do you have indigestion or heartburn? ☐

9. Do you have abnormal bodily reactions to alcohol such as flushing, headache, sinus congestion or itchy skin? ☐

10. Do you crave sugar or wheat products? ☐

11. Do you have fatigue? ☐

12. Do you feel lethargic? ☐

13. Do you have difficulty concentrating? ☐

14. Do you have depressed moods? ☐

15. Do you have allergy symptoms? ☐

16. Do you have recurrent respiratory infections? ☐

17. Do you have joint pain? ☐

18. Do you have muscle pain? ☐

Total Score – Add up your 'yes' answers

< 10   – It is not likely that you have yeast overgrowth

10–15 – Yeast overgrowth is a definite possibility

> 15   – Yeast overgrowth is very likely

LOW TESTOSTERONE
QUESTIONAIRE

Read each question carefully and check the box if it applies to you. When you finish calculate your score.

1. Do you have fatigue or low energy? ☐
2. Do you have a lack of drive? ☐
3. Do you lack initiative? ☐
4. Are you less assertive? ☐
5. Do you have a decline in your sense of well being? ☐
6. Do you have depressed moods? ☐
7. Are you frequently irritable? ☐
8. Has your self-confidence declined? ☐
9. Do you find it difficult to set goals? ☐
10. Do you have a difficult time making decisions? ☐
11. Have you had a decline in your mental sharpness? ☐
12. Has your vitality and endurance lessened? ☐
13. Have you lost muscle mass, strength or tone? ☐
14. Have you gained body fat around your waist? ☐
15. Do you have elevated cholesterol? ☐
16. Has your libido decreased? ☐
17. Has your sexual ability declined? ☐
18. Is it difficult to obtain or maintain an erection? ☐

Total Score – Add up all your 'yes' answers

< 7   – It is not likely that you have low testosterone
7–14   – Low testosterone is a possibility
> 14   – Low testosterone is very likely

SOME TERMS USED IN THIS BOOK

- **Adrenal glands**

  Organs that sit on top of the kidneys. They are chiefly responsible for regulating the stress response through the production of stress hormones, like cortisol and adrenaline.

- **Antioxidant**

  A molecule capable of slowing or preventing the oxidation of other molecules. Oxidation can produce free radicals that damage cells. Antioxidants stop this damage by removing free radicals. Thus, antioxidants are substances that may protect your cells against the effects of free radicals.

- **Cellular Nutrition Program**

  A patented nutritional supplement plan created, manufactured and distributed by Herbalife International. The basic program consists of three elements – a meal replacement shake drink, a multivitamin tablet and a herbal capsule. In simple terms, the shake and vitamin tablet provide all the key ingredients for balanced human nutrition while the capsule (called Cell Activator) optimises the absorption and utilisation of the nutrients at a cellular level.

- **CT (computerised tomography) scan**

  A special kind of X-ray investigation that provides far more details than ordinary X-rays. Instead of sending out a single X-ray through your body as with ordinary X-rays, several beams are sent simultaneously from different angles. A computer processes the results to create a picture shown on a monitor. CT scans have allowed doctors to inspect the inside of the body without having to operate or perform unpleasant examinations.

- **Excitotoxins**

  Chemicals that have a toxic stimulating effect on the nervous system. Some common foods and food additives have excitotoxin activity.

- **Free radical**

  Unstable chemical entities that readily react with and damage delicate substances and structures in the body. Some free radicals arise during the body's normal metabolism. Sometimes the body's immune system's cells purposefully create them to neutralise viruses and bacteria. However, environmental factors such as unhealthy food, pollution, radiation, cigarette smoke and herbicides can also spawn free radicals.

  Normally, the body can handle free radicals, but if antioxidants are unavailable, or if the free radical production becomes excessive, damage can occur. Of particular importance is that free radical damage accumulates with age and with many diseases.

- **Herb**

  Any plant with leaves, seeds, or flowers used for food, medicine, flavouring, or perfume.

- **IU**

  An abbreviation for **International unit** (from French *unité internationale*). It is a unit of measurement for the amount of a substance and is used for some vitamins, hormones, drugs, vaccines and similar biologically active substances.

- **Mineral**

  An inorganic substance needed by the human body for good health.

- **MRI (magnetic resonance imaging)**

  A newer technique than the CT scan. The MRI scan uses magnetic and radio waves, meaning that there is no exposure to X-rays or any other damaging forms of radiation. With an MRI scan it is possible to take pictures from almost every angle, whereas a CT scan only shows pictures in one plane. MRI scans are generally more detailed and the difference between normal and abnormal tissue is clearer.

- **ShapeWorks**

  ShapeWorks is a patented weight loss program manufactured by Herbalife International. It was developed by Dr David Heber, the Director of the Centre for Human Nutrition, UCLA. It customises your weight loss program based on your own body composition.

- **Stevia**

  Herb native to Paraguay whose leaves are the source of a non-caloric sweetener. It is available as a food supplement and is used as a sugar free sweetener.

- **Soy protein concentrate**

  Soy protein concentrate is made from defatted soybeans but, in addition to soy protein, it also contains much of the carbohydrates in the soybean. It contains about 65 per cent protein.

- **Soy protein isolate**

  Soy protein isolate is the purest form of soy protein available. It is made from defatted soybeans with almost all other ingredients removed. It contains 90+ per cent protein.

- **Supplement**

  A substance taken to remedy the deficiencies in a person's diet, for example, multivitamin supplements.

- **Textured soy protein**

  Textured soy protein is manufactured from soy protein concentrate and may be made to resemble various meat products such as beef, pork or chicken.

- **Vitamin**

  A group of organic compounds essential for normal growth and nutrition. They are essential in the diet because they cannot be made by the body.

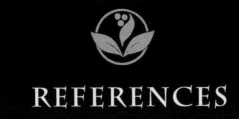

REFERENCES

BOOKS

The Wisdom of Menopause – Dr Christine Northrup

The LA Shape Diet – Dr David Heber

Born to be Healthy and Thin – Dr Steve Komadina

Natural Progesterone – Dr John Lee

What your Doctor may not tell you about Premenopause – Dr John Lee

How to Prevent Breast Cancer – Drs R. Pelton, C. Pelton & V. Wint

The China Study – Drs T. C. Campbell, T. M. Campbell

INTERNET SOURCES

Vendryes Wellness Centre – www.anounceofprevention.org

Life Extension Foundation – www.lef.org

News Target Insider Newsletter – www.NewsTarget.com

Mercola Newsletter –www.mercola.com

Townsend Letter – www.tldp.com

John R. Lee Newsletter – www.johnleemd.com

Herbalife International – www.herbalife.com

Treating Your Endometriosis – Dr Shelley Ross, e-book – www.treatendometriosis.com

Dr Nancy Dunne *PCOS Newsletter* – www.ovarian-cysts-pcos.com

5741911R00171

Printed in Great Britain
by Amazon.co.uk, Ltd.,
Marston Gate.